Copyright © 2015 Written, Designed and Created by Nicole White - www.NicoleWhiteWellness.com
Copyright © 2015 Illustrations and Design by Ayu Othman - www.ayuart.com

Published by: Nicole White Wellness
Nicole White
PO Box 31112
Santa Fe, NM 87594 (USA)

ISBN 10: 0990981614
ISBN 13: 978-0-9909816-1-9

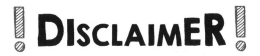

! DISCLAIMER !

The information in this book is for educational purposes only and should not be construed as medical advice. It is meant to supplement, not replace, any professional medical advice.

If you are on any medications or have a potential medical problem, it is imperative to seek the advice of a doctor or health care practitioner before making any dietary or lifestyle changes suggested in this book. While all information is based on scientific evidence, it is your responsibility to confirm with a medical professional that you may follow it without affecting your health. My publisher and I may not be held at fault for any injury that occurs as result of not consulting with a physician.

I urge you to do your research. You are the expert of your health and body. All of the suggestions in this book are merely that—suggestions! Use your best judgment and do not endanger your health. I truly believe that if you embrace and follow these simple upgrades you will see improvement to your health. Just make sure you check with a doctor before you begin.

All rights reserved. This book is for your use. All copyright rules apply. Please contact me directly if you would like to utilize this information as part of your personal project.

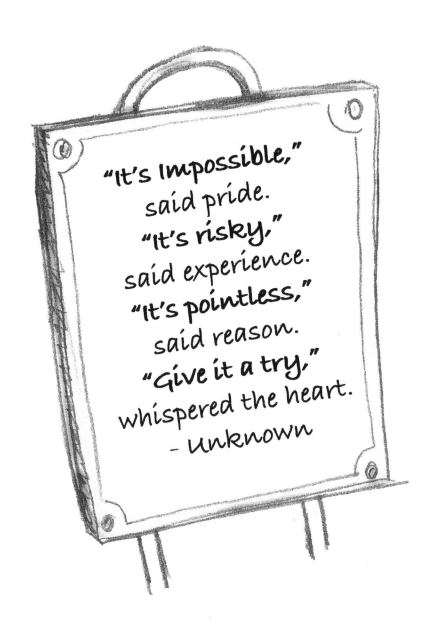

"It's Impossible,"
said pride.
"It's risky,"
said experience.
"It's pointless,"
said reason.
"Give it a try,"
whispered the heart.
- Unknown

Upgradeology is dedicated to Alan and Lynda White

Thank you both for believing in me, supporting me, and for all of your love and encouragement. I am forever grateful! Thanks for putting the "FUN in dysFUNctional." I love you SO much!

Huge GRATITUDE

To complete Upgradeology, I reached out to family and friends for their support. I would like to express a warm **Thank You** to everyone who contributed and believed in Upgradeology.

Alan & Lynda White	Valaphorn Tukovinit
Jacob & Bridgette White	Doris Hernandez McGinnis
Ryan & Genevieve White	Francois Houle
Mike & Bonny White	Luigi Dulanto
Gabriel & Anne White	Phebe Phillips & Mac Hargrove
Dustin White	Amorn Kittichartphayak
Mark Mason	Spencer Feix
Leslie Martin	Holly Willis
Valaluck Tukovinit	Kate OBinns

To the wonderful people whose loving emotional support has helped see this book through to completion.
Writing this book was a very isolating and difficult process. Every e-mail, phone call or get-together with an encouraging person helped me to re-fuel and re-commit.

Alan & Lynda White	Jacob White	Mel Mason
Avi Segal	Jenny Anthill	Michael White
Ayu Othman	Julia Catron	Phebe Phillips
Beth Lee	Kathleen Torres	Shalvah Orah
Cheri Anderson	Kim White	Sonette Steyn
Doris Hernandez-McGinnis	Leslie Martin	Tara Gesling
Harmony Rose West	Linda Barney	Val Tukovinit
Heathar Shepard	Mark Mason	Wade Knight
Holly Willis	Matthew Jager	Wendy Croze

Additional Gratitude

Thank you Dr. Arti Prasad, Michelle Hale and the University of New Mexico's Center for Life and Continuing Education facilities. Thank you for supporting and hosting my programs. You are the seed from which Upgradeology sprouted! Thank you Therese Pope for your editorial contribution! Thanks to anyone I forgot to include here, and to all of my teachers, guides, luck and obstacles along the way! Namaste.

A very special thank you to **Ayu Othman** for your **beautiful Illustrations!** I've wanted to collaborate with you for so long and I'm grateful that we have finally done it! You are an amazing woman, artist and friend! I admire and AYUpreciate your strength, determination, adventurous spirit and your beautiful skill and artistry. **YOU are such a Gift!**

INTRODUCTION

Does your mind **ping-pong** between the following?

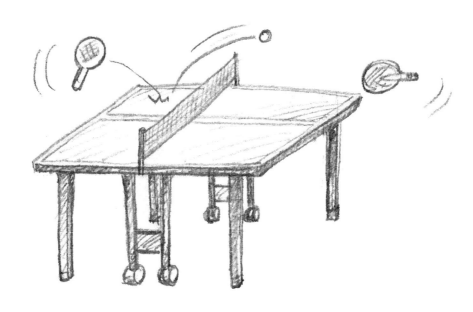

No meat - All meat

No carbS - Yes carbS

No gluten - Yes gluten

Low fat - High fat

No dairY - Yes dairY

Starve myself - Gorge myself

What if you could STOP looking for the next diet and BEGIN to honor and understand your food habits and cravings - by simply UPGRADING the Foods YOU Love?

When dieting, how many times have you fallen off the wagon?

Do you feel even worse because you give into your craving and reach for your old comfort foods? By gradually Upgrading the foods you crave with healthier versions of your favorite food or beverage, you will start to notice how much better you feel.

In this book, I give you **do-able steps** and tools to show you how to eliminate cravings for the foods that affect you negatively. I will help you incorporate clean, nourishing and SATISFYING foods into your daily life. Take the foods you LOVE and learn how to UPGRADE them with nourishing, clean ingredients that still satisfy your cravings, habits and lifestyle.

Think about the last time you ate a high-quality meal made with fresh, natural and organic ingredients, or enjoyed a favorite home-cooked meal. Maybe you remember walking into a restaurant or friend's home and were greeted with the sumptuous smells of wholesome comfort food. Did you rave to your friends and family about how delicious the food tasted? Did you remember the fresh ingredients and rich, beautiful colors and textures of the food? Nothing tastes better than a delicious, made-from-scratch meal prepared with clean, real and nourishing ingredients.

After this meal, did you wonder how you could **replicate this same amazing food experience at home?**

Why Upgrade to Real, Nourishing Food?

Food can be both healthy AND delicious. Processed foods desensitize you from being able to enjoy the taste of real foods. As a result, you may have to re-train your taste buds to recognize and enjoy the taste of real food again. It's extremely important that you ENJOY your food in order to keep eating it. This is why you can't stick to THAT diet: you don't enjoy the diet because the food just doesn't taste good to you.

Before processed foods became popular, people ate really clean and healing food. There was a time when produce was not sprayed with pesticides and herbicides. Master gardeners knew how to plant various crops in order to naturally ward off pests. Livestock was not constrained to an indoor factory or in a cage it could not move in, and pumped full of hormones and antibiotics. Livestock had room to roam and eat, and they had fresh air and a quality life outdoors. Most livestock are now born and raised in a factory, some never see the light of day, and they are fed grain and corn because it's cheap and fattens them up quickly.

Introduction

Because food has been so altered from its original state, your taste buds are confused from the toxic overload of chemical and flavor enhancers. As a result, most people don't remember how amazing real foods taste anymore. We expect food to be cheap, quick, and to taste exactly the same every time we purchase it.

The toxicity of chemically processed foods may create undesirable symptoms in your body. Unnatural food-like substances (a.k.a. frankenfoods) can aggravate and contribute to a range of common illnesses and diseases:

* **Exhaustion & Fatigue**
* **Anxiety & Depression**
* **Acid Reflux**
* **Hormonal Issues**
* **Brain-Fog**

* **Headaches**
* **Gut Issues & Bloating**
* **Inflammation & Joint Pain**
* **Insomnia/Sleep Issues**
* **Diabetes**

In the following chapters, I present a **DO-able,** livable food action plan that **encourages** you to **eat the food you love** and enjoy while enhancing your health and healing.

How to use Upgradeology

There is NOT just ONE way to eat for everyone, as we each have a deeply personal and emotional connection with the foods we love and crave. As you read through the chapters, you will notice that I don't lecture about restrictive dieting, counting calories, or avoiding fats or carbs. By restricting certain foods, you may think you are being "good" but that only lasts until you have an insatiable craving and desperately want that 'forbidden food' again. Instead of eating just one special treat, you find yourself gorging on it like you have been starved for days. Why did this happen again? Often, because you felt deprived.

As a Holistic Health Coach with training in Integrative Nutrition, I use the term "Upgrade" with private clients and the group courses I teach through the University of New Mexico's Center for Life and continuing education programs. Upgrading to healthier food leads you to make healing changes that become a way of life and not just another fad diet. Through my own food trial and errors and working with clients, I learned that eating healthy and focusing on the QUALITY, not the quantity, of your food creates long-lasting results. Healthy food doesn't have to be bland and tasteless. Who wants to eat blah food that has the texture of puffed cardboard? Yuck!

Before working together, many of my clients had difficulty switching over to a natural way of eating. They attempted numerous diets but always felt deprived and hopeless, then gave up out of frustration. I teach them a new way to approach their relationship with food. I show them how to read food ingredients and understand the difference between "real" food (fresh, natural and nourishing) versus "fake" (chemically-processed, mood-altering, inflammation and disease promoting) food-like substances. I also encourage my clients to become friendly with their kitchen. They are often surprised and delighted by the tasty treats they create out of "healthy foods" - without sacrificing their cravings or giving up foods they love.

With any new process, my clients realize that it takes time to create a new ritual around food. By helping you take small incremental steps, even though it may seem like the slow train, you will arrive there faster because you aren't waiting for that "perfect" moment to jump into action. Let's put a halt to the perfectionism that holds you back from achieving what you truly desire with your health goals! You can release perfectionism by embracing the baby step approach of the slow and steady Upgrade process.

You may ask yourself: how do I take that next step and transition to cleaner eating which creates greater health and well-being? The habits that hindered your health were set in place over time. Because these habits didn't happen overnight, it takes time and patience to cultivate new, lasting rituals that benefit the shift to eating for your healthiest self.

When confronted with your current health issues, do you tell yourself that "it isn't that bad?" Then say to yourself you will begin tomorrow, but tomorrow keeps getting put off. In this book, I will show you how to let go of that "all or nothing" mentality. You will learn how to incorporate easy and effective ways to create better health - without having to heave on board that next, new, promises-you-the-world diet. Use these baby steps in a way that works best with YOUR personal lifestyle.

Whether this is the beginning or continuation of your healing journey, welcome! I don't believe in the "one-size-fits-all "diet approach. **If diets really worked, you would not seek better information. I encourage you to move towards the suggestions that feel right to you. Then tweak and alter them to suit your lifestyle. Small positive shifts create long lasting results and healing over time.**

Here is what one client has to say about the Upgrading process:

"When Nicole taught me how to 'upgrade' my food, I was amazed at the difference it made in how my food tastes and how I feel! I was so excited about the promising changes I saw happening with me. I can't possibly say how much Nicole's non-judgmental approach, broad range of coaching skills and tools, and generous support, encouragement and guidance has focused my own efforts and given me confidence that I truly can make permanent, healthy changes that I hope will ultimately lead to life-changing transformation." - Holly, Albuquerque, NM

1 Baby-Stepology

Why Diet's Don't Work

The Baby Step Approach...13

Endless Curiosity..15

Why the Upgrade Process Works...16

Gratitude...18

How to Set Goals...20

Satisfaction Chart...21

Symptoms...24

Add-Ins / Upgrades...28

2 Craveology

Understand Your Food Cravings & Their Messages

Why Willpower Alone May Not Work..35

Honor Your Cravings / Purple Unicorn...36

Patterns and Possibilities for Cravings 37

Common Underlying Causes of Cravings 38

How Cravings Connect Us to Our Past...40

What are the Ingredients 41

What Do You Feel When You Have Food Cravings 42

Upgrade Your Cravings 44

Water 46

3 Ingredientology

The Importance of Reading Ingredients

Ingredientology is Simple..53

Don't Judge a Product by it's Nutritional Facts..............................54

Become an Ingredientologist 55

Organics...56

Organic Shopping Tips 57

How to Understand Produce Labels & Stickers 58

Nourishing Foods...59

Cholesterol and it's Bad Rap...60

Fill Up Faster and Stay Satisfied 64

4 Sweetology & Frankenology

Understand What's In YOUR Food

Sugar 67

Side Effects of Refined Sugar 68

Sugar and the Dangers of Food Marketing 69

Processed and Packaged Foods (Frankenfoods) 70

Symptoms That Could Be Related To Refined Sugars? 71

The Scary on Artificial Sweeteners - Frankenfoods 73

Not-So-Sweet Effects of Artificial Sweeteners 74

How to Upgrade from Artificial Sweeteners 75

How to Detox from Sugar Without Biting Off Someone's Head..... 76

Upgrades for Refined Sugar & Artificial Sweeteners 77

The Banana VS the Pancake 81

What are Frankenfoods? 82

UPGRADED SWEETENERS 83

Questionable Sweeteners 86

Toxic and Fake Food-Like Stuff 88

UPGRADES from Frankenfoods 88

How to Upgrade from Toxic and Artificial Frankenfoods 97

5 Blood-Sugarology

Food Combo's to Harmonize Mood & Stabilize Blood Sugar

Magic Trio Combination 101

Fiber, Protein and Fat 104

It's All About the Sauce 106

How to Create Your Own Sauces & Spreads 108

Release the Diet Mentality 110

Nourishing Fats 111

Breakfast 112

Snacks & Blood Sugar Stabilization 114

Fast Carbs, Slow Carbs & Fruit Carbs 116

"Gotta Go Bag" 118

Enzymes 120

Probiotic Foods 122

Understand Your Food, Understand Your Mood 126

6 Upgradeology

How to Satisfy Your Cravings with the Upgrade Process

Easy Upgrades to Get You Started 131
Upgrade Options 132
Breakfast Foods 133
Protein Shakes & Dairy 134
Meals & Snacks 136
Condiments, Condiments, Condiments 138
Make Your Own Dressing Chart 140
Beverages & Upgrade Chart 142
Caffeine - Quirky or Perky 144
10 Day NO-Withdrawl From Coffee Example 145
Recipe Alterations 150
Ingredient Conversions 152
Portion Control 157
How to Upgrade Your Family & Get Them on Board 157
Breakfast Options 158

7 Healingology

Learn How To Increase Energy With Nourishing Foods

Index of Healing Foods 161
How to Boost Your Energy With Fruit Juices/Smoothies 178
Energizing Drink - Fresh Green Juice 179

8 Successology

Shopping & Cooking Strategies For Successful Upgrading

I CAN List 181
How to Grow Your Own Sprouts 184
How to Prepare Frozen Meals 184
Cooking Hints 185
The WHY Upgrade List 186
Helpful Organic Shopping Tips 187
Going Out - Your Third Place 187
How To Get Organized 188
Kitchen Sanctuary 189

Food & Produce Prep Guide 191
Parasites 192
Cookware 192
Food Plan 194
Breakfast Options 195
Lunch & Dinner Options 196
Snack Options 198
Keep it Simple! 199

9 Wellnessology

Tips for Whole Body Wellness

You ARE That Magic Pill! 201
Restful Sleep Rituals 201
Write It Down to Figure It Out 204
Stress Relief 207
Meditation & Moving Meditation 208
Stretch Breaks & Gentle Yoga 209
Passion 211
Shake, Scream, Laugh & Sing 213
Gratitude 216
Movement & Exercise 216
Simple No - Equipment Exercises 218
Movement Worries 218
Weight Release & Self Talk 220
Blood Sugar Stabilization 222
How to Eat: Chewing & Digestion 223
Prepare For Eating 224
Sugar and Food Addiction 236

9.5 Summary

Baby Steps

Summary of Baby Steps 228
Recipes 230
Appendix 264
Index 266
Testimonials 272
About Nicole White & Ayu Othman 273

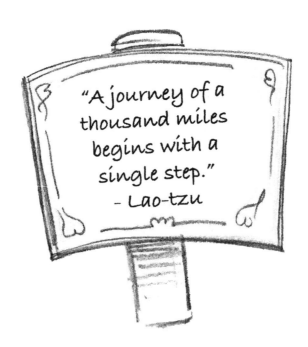

"A journey of a thousand miles begins with a single step."
– Lao-tzu

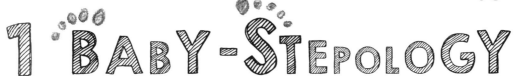

1 BABY-STEPOLOGY

Why Diet's Don't Work

The Baby Step Approach

What happens when you first start a new diet? Do you get really excited, jump into it head first, and try to do everything all at once? How many times have you dumped that new diet because you quickly became overwhelmed by it? Not to mention, you felt you couldn't do everything perfectly which made you feel worse and then possibly gave up altogether. You believe that if you can't do it perfectly then why bother. This is the 'all or nothing' mentality. The search for that perfect diet that usually ends up disappointing you…again.

This first chapter is about **giving you permission to move forward slowly and leave the diet mentality behind**. In order to take that first step, let's set that idea of perfectionism aside. Allow yourself to do it any way you can, and just take one little step at a time. For many people, perfectionism can keep you from even starting. I know this has been true for me and many of my clients.

So how can you take that first baby step? Use this book as an encouraging reference guide. First, flip through the chapters and see what feels comfortable as your first step. Then keep coming back to see what your next step will be. Or if something slips away, come back, re-commit, and take that small step again.

If you need help, the Baby Step exercises at the end of each chapter give you a nudge in the right direction! Remember you don't have to follow any particular order with these baby steps. Make it work for you and do it your own way. Take one little baby step at a time. **Every change, shift, or start in a positive direction WILL help you achieve long-term success.** Not doing something at all, because you believe you can't do it perfectly, can keep you from accomplishing the goals. So let the healing journey begin! Yes?

When you think of baby steps, what comes to mind?

What are one or two little things you could do that would eventually make a big difference in your life?

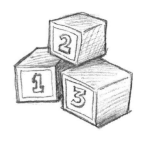

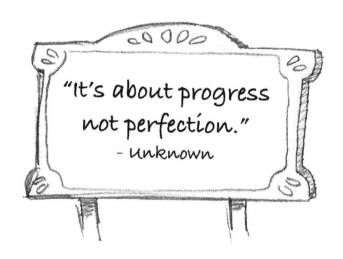

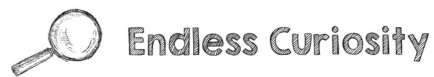

Endless Curiosity

My intent with this book is to share and encourage your new healing processes and reveal the ones that are harmful. I'm not asking you to believe me, or take my word for anything in this book. Instead, I offer information that has worked for me, worked for members in my programs, and for my private clients. I welcome you to conduct the research and see what works for you. So try it on for size and see if it fits. Does it need some alterations? If so, you are the tailor and you have the tools needed to make the information in this book fit your lifestyle needs and desires.

I welcome and encourage you to find the steps that work for you. For instance: most people know the dangers of artificial/chemical ingredients but some do not. If you take a chemical that has been known to harm people and look up the manufacturer of the product, they describe all the benefits but don't include the side-effects, or it's in some tiny fine print somewhere. They show a pretty picture of the product, show a fit, happy person consuming or holding the product, and make claims that the product is fat-free, calorie-free and diet friendly. However, they leave out the potentially harmful side effects. If you don't research, then you just take their word for it that you will be that thin, happy person IF you consume their products. That is the power of advertising.

I will teach you how to be curious. Let this book be your process of endless curiosity. I will show you how to look at what is really going on with food manufacturers, and what you are being led to consume. I hope that the information shared here makes you curious about the foods and substances you ingest, and how they either benefit or harm you.

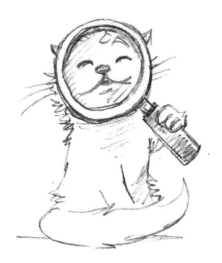

Why The Upgrade Process Works

Have you been round and round the different diet blocks? Have you ever clung to a 'diet' or a certain food lifestyle like it was your religion? There are many different concepts as to what makes up the healthiest diet and food plan. However, the foods that I eat may not work for someone else, and what works great for someone else won't necessarily work for me. As we change over time so do our needs. The suggestions outlined in the following chapters are your foundation for a more nourishing lifestyle. Find out what does and does not work for you, then tweak and adjust as necessary. "Give a man a fish and he eats for the day; teach him to fish and he eats for a lifetime." Let's learn to fish! AND because I honor all people and their choice to eat or not to eat fish…"Give a gal a salad and she eats for a day; teach her to garden and she eats for a lifetime." So let's get into the garden! (No worries, no dirt required here!)

Learn to Upgrade from processed, packaged, microwaved or denatured food-like substances. All true nourishing eating plans are sourced from nature. They all have a component of being plant-based from real, true, organic and clean sources. I see this as the agreeance so let's at least kumbaya about what we do agree with! I'm not suggesting that you follow a specific food plan such as vegan/vegetarian/paleo (among a large variety of options). **Only you know what foods feel best in your body and give you the energy and clarity you seek.**

There is a movie called "May I Be Frank" about a guy (Frank), who went from being almost 300 lbs on a variety of medications eating the SAD (Standard American Diet), to eating a mainly raw, vegan diet. Through his process, with quite the support system, he released about 140 lbs, released medications, and healed a slew of illnesses. As a result, he regained his health and zest for life. Frank mentioned he ate a lot of raw and plant based foods and then, with hesitation, he admitted to eating some animal products. I think there was a sneer, boo, hiss, shock throughout the mostly vegan audience when he said this. He chuckled embarrassingly and said it was harder to admit that he ate some chicken now and then than it was to admit that he was a former heroin addict.

I thought Frank's statement was brilliant. At the time I watched the movie, I was a hard-core raw vegan. Despite creating a vegan cookbook and centering the first few programs I taught on plant-based eating, I did my best not to preach this way of eating. I never told anyone that they had to be vegan… at least, I hope not. And if I did, I apologize for that.

Many people (like me) will dive in and adopt being (enter your food religion here) vegan, vegetarian, raw, paleo, and so on. Some people are confident that they need animal products for energy, nutrients and protein, while others feel that they thrive on a pure plant-based food plan. I want to create harmony within these pages for people in their own unique walks of life. I don't want someone to feel judged because they feel they 'should' be vegan - just as I wouldn't want a vegan to open a book promoting all animal products. People will do what they want and think what they think, and really that's none of my business. But since I've adopted many different food styles at different times of my life, I think it's fair and honest to create an all-inclusive, well-being book. When we convince ourselves that OUR way is the only way, we block out other possibilities that could lead to greater health and well-being.

I encourage you to go about this book (and your life) with endless curiosity, and to see how the pieces fit together for your unique life and well-being. Too often (think media's influence or 'keeping up with the Jones') **we 'think' we should be this or we shouldn't be that**. Tony Robbins says it perfectly "*Stop SHOULDing all over yourself.*" Believe in being yourself and you will live a far more fulfilled life! "*No one will ever be as good as you at BEING YOU.*"

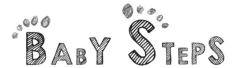

 **Write down a few things that you are 'stuck in your ways' about.**
This could be related to food, general health, world views, work issues, or anything that comes to mind:

 **What would it look like to become curious about this 'thing'? Write down the possible scenarios:**

 **Talk to someone who may have a different viewpoint or opinion about this topic.** Go into it with an open mind. You are there to learn and be curious instead of prove your point. Even if you are correct, is there something that you can learn from this other viewpoint?

Gratitude

Although it may seem like an unusual thing to say, I feel grateful for my past illnesses. If I had not gone through a variety of health problems, I would not have made significant changes to a healthier and more nurturing way of life. I'm glad that I found ways to heal myself naturally. It has been a long journey but a successful one, and it still continues. Because of these experiences and my positive results, I can now help others who suffer from chronic illnesses and food addiction. You may be unaware, just as I was, of how you can live your life to the fullest. It fills me with joy to be able to share my experiences with you.

Your decision to take action is a step along the path to naturally improve your health and well-being. Positive thinking keeps a bright picture in mind which helps you reach your vision and goals. As your guide on this journey, I provide you with information that will enable you to make the best decisions for YOUR health by making positive shifts with your food and emotional well-being.

Please read and understand the disclaimer: I am not a doctor and the advice of a medical professional should never be disregarded or solely replaced by the suggestions in this book.

There is a great deal of information in Upgradeology. Again, I encourage you to go at your own pace. Every little change, shift, and new ritual are helpful. You will begin to notice a positive difference in how you feel and move in the world. Doing the best you can is a change for the better that will have positive, lasting effects on your health.

It's a fact... the more you are grateful and thankful for, the more there is to be thankful and grateful for in your life. The more you complain and pay attention to what's going wrong…then it's more likely that more negative things will show up in your life. This isn't always easy. First, look around and feel gratitude for what you DO have. Chances are the computer you use, the clothing you wear, and the car you drive are all things you once wanted...and now you have them.

Gratitude has a chance to cultivate when you surround yourself with positive people and positive reinforcement. The news is all about fear so I recommend that you watch less of it or better yet, consider turning it off. Allow yourself to see what IS going well with the world. I realize this is MUCH easier SAID than done, but this too is a seed of possibility you may want to consider planting.

Knowledge without action won't nourish and grow the seeds you've just planted. It helps to KNOW what you are doing so you understand what steps to take. It's my goal to give you this information so you can take positive action steps forward. This can be as simple as creating a desire list that you look at often. Throughout this book, please take the time to jot down what you've discovered. This knowledge is the water that nourishes your recently planted seeds that need daily attention to grow and thrive!

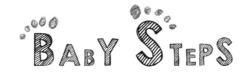

What are you GRATEFUL for?

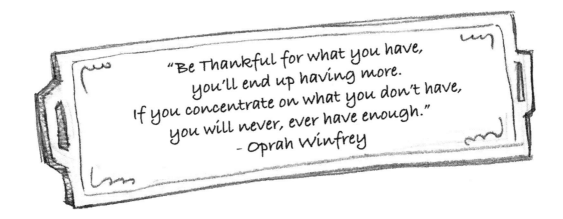

"Be Thankful for what you have,
you'll end up having more.
If you concentrate on what you don't have,
you will never, ever have enough."
- Oprah Winfrey

How To Set Goals

I rebelled against what was good for me because of childhood traumas, and because I just didn't want to be like my family. I threw out the good habits with the bad. Do you rebel at the expense of your own health? I was taught at a young age to write out the things that I wanted. Instead, I wrote about things that I felt were going wrong in my life. Guess what happened? I had more things to write about that were going wrong. When I started to write out my goals and create action steps for each goal, something magical happened. My goals became reality. Why? Because they were no longer lofty goals I dreamt about. They were things I achieved by writing out action steps and then taking baby steps towards each goal.

 First, think about your goals.
Write them here:

 Now think about what you rebel against in your life.
Write them here:

 Why do you rebel against things you know are 'good for you'?
Such as eating nourishing foods or getting appropriate movement for your body/lifestyle etc.? What are your reasons?

Dig into those childhood memories or past hurts/injuries and I'm sure you will find your rebellious reasoning. For example, when I was a kid my brothers and I had to clean our rooms 'perfectly' and vacuum EVERY DAY (not exaggerating) before leaving for school. The vacuum lines had to be 'just so'. Guess what happened when I got my first apartment? I resisted getting a vacuum! Guess what happened when they asked me to vacuum at work? I nearly lost a job because I kept resisting to vacuum when it was my turn.

Another example: My mother didn't want me to have 'weight issues' like she did as a kid so she put me on a diet. I only began to binge eat once I was put on that diet. As a child, it seemed unfair that the foods my brothers ate were off limits to me. So I began to sneak into the pantry at night and have my fill. Still to this day when I think about dieting, my first reaction is to binge eat.

What does this have to do with your goals? If they are health goals, there just may be a reason **why** you rebel against your own health. This is a good place to start figuring out **where and how you rebel**. Then take little baby steps towards creating a groove in your new path that feels good and that **YOU** enjoy!

20

Take the time to write this out now:

❓ **What are your health goals?**

❓ **What obstacles are in the way of achieving your health goals?**

❓ **Do you rebel against certain things that you KNOW are 'good for you'?**
   If so, what are the rebellions and what are the underlying reasons for them?

Notice the Satisfaction Chart below. Use this chart to see where you are in and out of harmony. Choose just one that is out of harmony, and then choose one you would like to focus on Upgrading now.

Satisfaction Chart

Note your satisfaction in the following areas: Scale of 1-5

1 = experience **LEAST** amount of satisfaction

5 = experiences the **MOST** amount of satisfaction

_____ **Sleep**	_____ **Career**
_____ **Finances**	_____ **Work Relationships**
_____ **Health**	_____ **Movement**
_____ **Weight**	_____ **Time in Nature**
_____ **Friends**	_____ **Passion/Hobbies**
_____ **Family**	_____ **Peace of Mind (Sleep and Wake easy)**
_____ **Home Life**	_____ **Spiritual Life (Community/Nature)**

Look at the above list, now put them in order of importance to you.

1._____   8. _____

2. _____   9. _____

3. _____   10. _____

4._____   11. _____

5. _____   12. _____

6. _____   13. _____

7. _____   14. _____

I - Baby-Stepology

Now, let's look at the places in your life that you ARE happy about. What are the top 3 that you ARE happy/content with?

1.   2.   3.

List out a few reasons WHY these are special to you and how to cultivate more of that in your life.

What are the 3 you would most like to work on, or you feel would most enhance your life?

1.   2.   3.

Then list 3 small baby action steps you can begin taking to help improve these areas. See examples below:

Examples:
Baby Step #1 - Passion

1. Take 5 minutes each day to paint, write, learn/play a musical instrument, research and so on.
2. Take 5 minutes every morning and night towards a passion/hobby.
3. Take 5 minutes every morning **AND** night, as well as dedicate one hour on weekends, to your hobby/passion – just going through the motions.

Baby Step #2 - Movement

1. Take a walk around the block before work every day, just 3-5 minutes.
2. Take a short walk around the block before work and then at lunch time, 5-7 minutes total.
3. Take a walk before work, at lunch, and after work, 10 minutes total.

Baby Step #3 - Eat nourishing ingredients

1. Make a list of trigger foods that are in your kitchen right now. A trigger food may be something that leads you to overeat or crave foods you've sworn off.
2. Set and write the date on your calendar for when you plan to clean out your kitchen of trigger foods.
3. Call a friend or ask someone you live with to help you with this project and have them take away the food.

Your Turn! List 3 small baby action steps for your top 3 categories:

Baby ACTION Step for _____

1.

2.

3.

Baby ACTION Step for _____

1.

2.

3.

Baby ACTION Step for _____

1.

2.

3.

Symptoms

"I have continued to keep processed sugar out of my food plan, including alcohol, and my weight has stabilized. My energy is higher and my pain level when walking has greatly decreased. These baby steps are something that I've newly included into my lifestyle. They have really enriched my life and improved my physical and mental health in the midst of a real health crisis. Thank you!" - Susan, New Mexico

An important part of the healing process is gradual improvement. In order to know what you have accomplished, you'll want a measurement of where you are now and where you want to be. So be honest when jotting down your symptoms.

What would it be like if you had less pain and more mobility to enjoy life?

Do you have any of the following symptoms?

Note the symptoms you experience and then look for the root cause of them. Many of these symptoms listed below are food and dehydration related.

- [ ] Headache
- [ ] Moodiness
- [ ] Irritability
- [ ] Road Rage
- [ ] Insomnia
- [ ] Achy Joints and Muscles
- [ ] Inflammation
- [ ] Back Pain
- [ ] Arthritis
- [ ] Rash
- [ ] Eczema
- [ ] Acne
- [ ] Lethargy
- [ ] Brain Fog
- [ ] Constipation

- [ ] Diarrhea
- [ ] Irritable Bowel Syndrome
- [ ] Crohn's
- [ ] Celiac
- [ ] Leaky Gut
- [ ] Stiff Neck and Shoulders
- [ ] Knots in your Stomach,
- [ ] Allergies
- [ ] Respiratory Issues
- [ ] Gout
- [ ] Acidity in Stomach or Esophagus
- [ ] Kidney Stones
- [ ] Diabetes
- [ ] Hypoglycemia
- [ ] Other _____

Use the Symptoms Chart to get clear about the symptoms you have.

Write down the symptoms that you want to release:

1.

2.

3.

What do you believe needs to happen to release these symptoms?
It's OK if you don't know yet!

1.

2.

3.

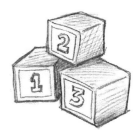 **What new ritual or healthy habit do you believe needs to be adopted in order to relieve yourself of unwanted symptoms?** This includes excess weight, fatigue, medications, skin issues, chronic illness, and so on?

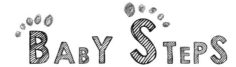

What is the biggest issue in your life right now that you want resolved: Write it here:

Write down 3 things that would help resolve that biggest issue.
Things that are SMALL (think little baby steps) and do-able this week:

1.

2.

3.

Pick just ONE Baby Action Step!
Get your calendar, and set a DATE and TIME to do it:

* If you put your action steps on the calendar and find that you aren't doing them, then this step is too big. Find an even smaller step and re-commit. Keep doing this until you are able to do the action step, and then decide your next step.

Example

Issue: Co-worker brings junk food to office, lays it out in communal space, and I have difficulty not eating it.

Resolution: Ask co-worker to put it in a more discreet place where you don't have to see it or ask him/her to leave it on their desk instead of in the lunch room.

Time to do this: Friday afternoon, 4pm.

What happened? Did not feel comfortable approaching coworker, afraid of his reaction.

Thought: I should be strong enough to be able to resist the temptation of that yummy- looking food as I have to pass by it 25 times a day. By now, I'm old enough that I should have more will power to just say no. I resolve to not let it get to me.

Monday Morning: I gave in… gosh - why am I so weak?

Re-commitment: I'm obviously having difficulty with the work treats placed in the break room and it would be better not to see them all day and be tempted. I resolve to bring in my own snacks, as well as commit to talking with co-worker on Tuesday morning before he lays out the treats.

What happened: Wow, I approached my coworker and his response was better than I thought. He apologized for bringing in the treats and was actually glad I said something. He was tired of having to fork out money for them and was a great excuse not to bring them in all the time. He just loves the interaction with people, so he decided to change and put a little bowl of treats on his desk. This way more people can stop by and say hi. What a great compromise! I'm glad we talked. I had a much better day because I was not as tempted by the treats. I ate all the snacks that I brought and felt really satisfied. Amazingly enough, I have more energy after work than I've felt in a very long time.

See Snacks (page 114) **for more information on how to navigate the office.**

Simple things to incorporate - **Add-Ins, page 28**

Headaches - **Water, page 46**

Sugar Cravings - **Cravings, page 35**

How to Eat Healthier - **Upgradeology, page 131**

Blood Sugar Issues - **Magic Trio Combinations, page 101**

Mood issues - **Food/Mood Journal, page 126**

Trouble shopping? - **I Can List, page 181**

Sweet Tooth - **Upgraded Sweeteners, page 77, 83-85**

Digestion & Gut Issues - **Enzymes & Probiotic Foods, page 120-123**

Trouble sleeping? - **Sleep, page 201**

Perfectionism? - **Baby Steps, page 13**

Night Eating/Binge Eating - **Breakfast and Snacks, page 112 & 114**

Food Temptations - **Purple Unicorn, page 36**

It CAN'T be MY food! - **Ingredientology, page 54 & 126**

Add-Ins/Upgrades

The moment you decide to stop eating your favorite food, do you then find yourself thinking about it even more? Have you ever declared that you were going to give something up AFTER you finish just... this...last...one? Are you waiting to find your favorite food on the 'forbidden food list'?

Don't know where to begin? Begin by adding in nutritional foods. It is MUCH easier to add in something new rather than take something old (and comforting) away.

As you start to experiment with add-ins and other nourishing "real food" Upgrades, keep a journal or notebook and track how you feel, your progress, and your struggles. Go ahead and write directly in this book, or create a journal or notebook to take notes about what's most important to you. Refer to Chapters 5 & 9 and learn how journaling can help you stay on track.

Since the Upgrade process is ALL about baby steps, start with these simple nutrients that you can easily begin to add into your meals and/or snacks. Start with just ONE that looks the most appealing to you.

See Chapters 5 and 6 for more Upgrades & Add-Ins

Organic Turmeric (Curcumin)

Benefits

* A natural antiseptic and antibacterial agent
* A natural liver detoxifier and pain killer
* May prevent or slow the progression of Alzheimer's
* Has been used in India as an anti-inflammatory treatment for arthritis and rheumatoid arthritis
* Used in China as treatment for depression
* Speeds up wound healing and helps with inflammatory skin conditions
* Anti-cancer and cancer-healing properties

Uses

* Add to food or drinks.
* Use in curries and stews.
* Heal pain and inflammation
* **Golden Milk Recipe** on page 236.

Organic Turmeric Powder

Organic Ceylon Cinnamon

Benefits

* May assist in lowering blood sugar
* Contains antioxidants
* Promotes healthy liver function
* Anti-inflammatory
* Anti-fungal properties
* Smelling can boost brain function
* Stabilizes blood sugar

Uses

* 1/4 tsp to 1-1/2 tsp **max** per day is recommended.
* It is delicious sprinkled on food such as apples or baked squash.
* Adds a natural sweetness to tea and drinks.

Don't overdo cinnamon, as it's NOT recommended in large doses.

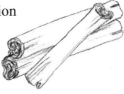

Organic Chia Seeds

Benefits

* 2 grams of protein per tablespoon
* 4 grams of fiber per tablespoon
* Contains Vitamin A, C, B1, B2, niacin, foliate, calcium, iron, phosphorous, magnesium, zinc, selenium, copper, manganese, and potassium
* Contains all 3 Omegas - Omega 3, 6 & 9
* Contains 18 essential amino acids unaltered (altered amino acids can sometimes be compromised)
* Double the amount of protein found in any grain
* 3 times the antioxidants of blueberries
* 3 times more iron than spinach
* Double the amount of potassium in a banana

Uses

* Chia seeds (when hydrated) have the consistency of tiny tapioca.
* Create puddings or gels out of them.
* Sprinkle them on top of your favorite foods or sauces to start.
* Blend with an avocado and your favorite Upgraded Sweetener (page 77, 83-85) to create pudding.
* Add Chia to a smoothie or sprinkle on your favorite breakfast food.

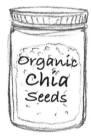

More Information

One to two tablespoons daily is all that is needed. Chia seeds have no taste. Sprinkle them on any food or mix in water. To use them, add water and stir. Set for one minute and then continue to stir so they don't clump to the bottom. They will expand to about nine times their original size. My favorite way to use them is to put them in water, and shake every few minutes until they float. Add some coconut sugar (or green stevia powder), cinnamon and goji berries. burning and it makes a delicious, portable and hydrating snack.

Breakfast Chia

* 1/2 cup of chia seeds
* 2 cups of almond or coconut milk
* 3-5 drops of vanilla stevia (or any Upgraded Sweeteners you like)
* 1/4 tsp cinnamon
* 1/2 cup raw mixed nuts (cashews, almonds, pecans, walnuts)
* Celtic Sea Salt to taste

Directions:

1. Blend chia seeds, milk, stevia, salt and cinnamon together.
2. Place in refrigerator overnight or for a couple of hours to thicken.
3. In the morning, add nuts and sea salt to taste.

To serve warm:
1. Place in a pot over LOW heat
2. Gently heat to about 110 degrees. Enjoy!

Organic Extra Virgin Coconut Oil

Benefits

* A feel-good food
* Loaded with good saturated fats and lauric acid, a powerful nutrient for immune system
* Natural antioxidant
* One of very few oils that are safe at high heat (if you fry, fry with coconut oil)
* Helps boost brain function - top recommended food to prevent Alzheimer's
* Helps increase energy and assists in burning fat

Uses

* Replace other cooking oils.
* Use for high-heat cooking such as baking or frying.
* Use in hot drinks to replace milk.
* Use instead of dairy as a thickener or to add moisture.
* Replace butter for vegan recipes.
* Can be used as natural skin moisturizer and sunscreen.

 I love to use coconut oil in my morning drinks. I use it as a thickener instead of milk. Try this warm, soothing Hot Chocolate Recipe below. It's a delicious and nourishing Upgrade from refined sugar or chemically-processed cocoa mixes.

Hot Chocolate (use organic whenever possible)

Ingredients

* 1 TBSP Raw Cacao Powder
* 1 TBSP Organic Extra Virgin Coconut Oil
* 1 TBSP Coconut Sugar
* 1 TBSP Maca (optional)
* 1/8 tsp Cinnamon
* 8-12 oz Purified Water
* Pinch of Celtic Sea Salt (to taste)

Directions

1. Add cacao powder, coconut sugar, maca, cinnamon and purified water into a blender.
2. Blend until smooth.
3. Pour mixture into a sauce pan, ADD coconut oil, and turn to medium high heat.
4. Heat until desired temperature and then pour into your favorite mug. Yum!

*Play around with the ingredients until it tastes just right for you:

Want it **thicker**? Add more coconut oil or coconut butter

Want it **thinner**? Add more warm/hot water

Want a **stronger chocolate flavor**? Add more cacao powder

Want it **sweeter**? Add more Upgraded sweetener (see Upgraded Sweeteners on pages 77, 83-85).

If you drink **coffee/lattes/ mochas,** consider buying **fair trade organic coffee beans** and make your own.

* You can add 8-12 oz organic coffee to the **Hot Chocolate Recipe** to make your own **Mocha**.
* For a **Latte**, just remove the cacao.
* For an **Americano**, add your favorite Upgraded Sweetener or drink as is.

Note: If you know your body doesn't do well with coffee see **Upgraded Beverages** on page 142 more options.

Organic RAW Apple Cider Vinegar

Benefits

* Aids in digestion
* Rich in enzymes and potassium
* Natural antibiotic
* Assists in reducing inflammation, and eases arthritis and stiffness
* Can also be used to heal the skin and as a hair rinse
* Removes toxins in the body
* Contains protein, enzymes, and good 'friendly' bacteria

Uses

* There are books written on the benefits and uses of Organic RAW Apple Cider Vinegar. (Look online for more benefits)
* 1 TBSP ACV (Apple Cider Vinegar)to 8-12 oz Purified water and drink before meals as a digestive aide.
* **Use instead of other vinegars for dressings and other vinegar-based sauces and foods.**
* Put on a cotton ball and use as deodorant.
* Create a brine for fermenting vegetables.

Raw Organic Apple Cider Vinegar – is the only vinegar I use. It's made by fermenting organic apples. You can even make it at home! It makes for a delicious tart dressing base, and can be used in tonic drinks. Always dilute Apple Cider Vinegar before drinking!

Apple Cider Vinegar Tonic Drink

* 8 oz purified water
* 1 TBSP Organic Raw Apple Cider Vinegar
* 1 tsp (to taste) local or truly raw honey (optional) or your favorite natural sweetener

Directions:

With a spoon, stir ingredients together in 8 oz glass.
Make sure honey and sweetener are dissolved before drinking.

Celtic Sea Salt & Himalayan Salt

Benefits

* Contains trace minerals that help hydrate
* Contains powerful electrolytes such as magnesium
* Contains trace elements that assist with adrenal, immune, and thyroid health
* Helps prevent muscle cramps
* Regulates sleep
* Alkalizes the body
* Balances blood sugar

Uses

* Add to any food to bring out more of it's natural flavor.

* Use in replacement of all table salts.

Table salt is full of stabilizers, and is stripped of nutrients. Table salt can contribute to ill health.

31

Organic Tea

Organic Green Tea

Benefits

* Loaded with antioxidants
* Has anti-anxiety effect (unlike coffee)
* More stable form of caffeine and energy
* Improves brain function
* Fat burning properties
* Reduces risk of cancer
* Can lower risk of viruses and infections

Uses

* Use green tea when you are trying to wean yourself off coffee, energy-drinks, black tea, or soda. Like most products, the cheap brands are chemically altered.
* Treat your body well and get yourself an organic brand.

Organic Peppermint Tea

Benefits

* Soothes and relieves digestive discomfort
* Cool and uplifting - sniff before drinking
* Calms an overactive stomach
* Can ease headaches

Uses

* Use as an after meal digestive aide.
* Use to ease pain.
* Use to relax the body and mind.

Organic Chamomile Tea

Benefits

* Best known as a natural sleep aid
* Relaxing and soothing
* An immune booster
* Relief for fevers or colds
* Can aid digestion after a meal
* Reduces inflammation

Uses

* Use instead of sleeping pills.
* Use to relax and calm naturally.
* See Warnings.

*WARNING: If you are allergic to the ragweed family (i.e. daisies, asters, chrysanthemums), be cautious about chamomile tea as you may find the same allergens. First, test a very small amount. If you have any negative reactions, discontinue use immediately. If you think you may be allergic or if you have never tried Chamomile tea, start by letting the teabag steep for just a few dips, then on the next cup steep longer (if you don't have negative side effects). Side effects may begin as a tingle in the back of the throat (or more) depending on your sensitivity.

NOTE: If you take any medications, or if you are pregnant or nursing, be sure to check with your doctor first before consuming any of the items listed above or in this book.

Which of these Add-Ins/Upgrades are you willing to try?

There is something powerful about writing things down on paper. How many times have you forgotten something important because you didn't write it down? Begin to write ideas down as you work your way through the Upgrade process. I've intentionally left space for you to write throughout this book.

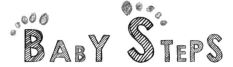

Write down the item that looks most appealing to you. Either put it on your shopping list or try it at your next meal or tea-time:

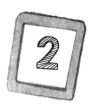

Once you are comfortable with the first step, write down another one to add in:

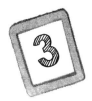

Now add a third item to experiment with:

In this first chapter we discussed:

* The Baby Step Approach
* Getting and staying curious
* Why the Upgrade process works
* How to increase your health and well-being with Gratitude
* The importance of setting do-able goals
* How to easily Add-In Upgraded ingredients

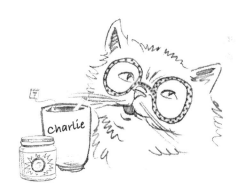

I hope you started to become curious about the foods you eat and how taking baby steps towards your health goals will get you there quicker. Consider where perfectionism gets in your way and which baby steps break through that barrier. Let's get curious and figure out why you crave certain foods (i.e. sweets, processed, refined or diet foods, etc.).

In Chapter 2, you will discover the hidden meanings behind your food cravings – i.e. why you crave refined sugars and processed foods and how they negatively impact your health. As you read, I encourage you to explore the Baby Steps at the end of each chapter. Become curious and adopt what works best for your personal lifestyle!

2 - Craveology

She spreads her love around freely
Even pays for it
Pays for all of them
To love her?
She looks outward
Seeing what out there will satisfy her

She walks the aisles
Scanning them up and down
Looking for that perfect lover
Of who can satisfy her tonight

She pays for it freely
Night after night
Letting them invade her body

Looking for love
In a different taste and texture
But never finding it there

Trying to shush the voices
As they drag back old memories
Where the only safety seemed to be
In the comfort of bottomless bowls

There is never enough
Night after night
There is never enough

And tomorrow's self promises
Are pushed off
Yet another day
Yet again

And if everything is for a reason
Then this is where she is
Parked at the market
Looking for love
Paying for it
And leaving

    Unsatisfied

2 CRAVEOLOGY
Understand Your Food Cravings & Their Hidden Messages
Why willpower alone may not work

You can talk about willpower all day long. You may get pumped up and motivated, start that new diet, and have every intention of complete commitment. You clean out every trace of junk food from the cabinet, and shout it from the rooftops: "No more (insert your poison here)!" But then you wake up in some kind of fog with that craved food package sitting empty in your hands. You cry and whimper like you have committed some vicious, inadvertent crime; you berate yourself for your "weakness." You repeat that self-delusional lie to yourself—that this is truly the last time—and make plans to really kick the habit tomorrow. . . next week . . . after the holidays . . . next year . . .

What are your tools when willpower fails you? What will keep you from repeating this pattern next time? You are told that there is always the standard line of defense: more self-help books; the next fad diet; the next anti-craving pill; and the new magic potion that will do the trick for good this time! It reminds me of a cartoon I once saw:

> A depressed man walks into a bookstore and asks the sales attendant, "Hi, where's the self-help section?"
>
> The attendant pauses a moment before responding and then says, "If I told you, it would defeat the purpose."

I mention this because it is essential to dispel the notion that every failure is a matter of willpower. What if every "failure" is an insight that leads you closer and closer to your own personal success? It's difficult for many of us to recognize anything but our failures so I ask you...

What would the world be like without some of these Famous Failures?

The Beatles - Their first record was rejected.

Oprah Winfrey - Was told she wasn't fit for television.

Albert Einstein - Teachers said he was stupid.

Walt Disney - Fired for not having any original ideas, lacking creativity.

Lucille Ball - Was told to find a different career by her drama teacher.

Michael Jordan - Thrown out of his high school basketball team.

Stephen Spielberg - Rejected from film school.

J.K. Rowling - Was a single mother on welfare when she wrote Harry Potter.

Thomas Edison - Made over 10,000 unsuccessful attempts before succeeding at inventing the light bulb.

So what if it's **not** about willpower? What if cravings are **messages** bubbling up to the surface in a language you don't **yet** understand?

35

Honor Your Cravings
Give Them The Attention They Want & Deserve

Let's take a moment and honor your cravings! Your body and mind are so amazing and fantastic. What if these cravings that you try to deny, fight, and finally give into are telling you something? What if they are telling you something really important?

Lean in…can you hear it? What is your body telling you? Do you crave certain foods when you are stressed? Certain foods when you feel lonely or misunderstood? Certain foods when you are angry, frustrated, and just wish you could…(enter your reactions here).

? What do your cravings tell you?

? What happens when you try to deny yourself one of your favorite foods?

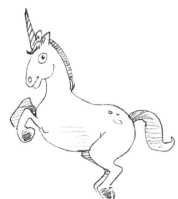

Try this exercise: I'm going to ask you **NOT** to think about a **Purple Unicorn**. Don't think about its **shape** or size or **magical powers**. Remember do NOT think about a Purple Unicorn. Whatever you do, DON'T think about the purple unicorn! Got it?

So…what are you thinking about? A purple unicorn, perhaps? This is the exact same scenario we use when we attempt to restrict ourselves from the foods we crave—we can't NOT think about them. In fact, we think about them even more!

Some questions to ask yourself the next time cravings comes on strong:

? Are you dehydrated? Have you had enough water today, or just caffeine, soda's and concentrated fruit juice?

? Are you hungry? Did you skip breakfast? Go too long without a snack? Has your blood sugar dropped to the point where you can't think straight until you eat something?

? Are emotions high? Angry, lonely, sad, anxious (fill in the blank) _____

? Are you stressed out? Taking on the weight of the world at home, work, relationships, finances, family?

Honor your emotions and you will begin to **understand** what your **cravings** are asking of you.

Take some time to think about your cravings and write your answer below.

? What do YOUR Cravings tell you?

Patterns and Possibilities for Cravings

There are many reasons why you crave particular food items. Here are a few: Check off the ones that may apply to you, even if some situations only occur once in a while. Check them off so that you can see what triggers your cravings.

Some possible reasons for cravings:

- [ ] **You still taste the food you just ate**
- [ ] **You see or think about a favorite childhood food**
- [ ] **Comfort Foods - Hearty foods that you think will make you feel more grounded**
- [ ] **Ancestry Foods - The foods your 'tribe' ate, foods connected with your culture**
- [ ] **The Void - Feeling alone or lethargic/frustrated with reality**
- [ ] **Emotions - Tired, wired, angry, lonely, bored, sad, frustrated, happy, disbelief, among other emotions**
- [ ] **Job/Career/Work - Too stressful or not fulfilling**
- [ ] **Nutrient Deficiencies - Eating mostly processed and refined foods/fast foods**
- [ ] **Hormones - Seasons/cycles - Hormones hidden in your foods**
- [ ] **Dehydration - Not having enough purified water or water-rich foods**
- [ ] **Seasons - Different cravings for different seasons**
- [ ] **Holidays - Obligations and expectations - surrounded by delicious looking foods**
- [ ] **Current events/Crisis in home life/work/community/country/world**
- [ ] **Relationships - New/Challenging or Old/Challenging**
- [ ] **Community - Do you lack your 'tribe' or are you involved in one that doesn't serve you?**
- [ ] **Blood Sugar - Do you go for long periods of time without eating and/or skip breakfast or lunch?**
- [ ] **Visual Triggers - TV, advertisements, other people's food, drive-thru**
- [ ] **Aromatic Triggers - The smell going past the bakery, other people's foods**
- [ ] **Lack of Movement - Stagnant energy and using food to stuff it down further**
- [ ] **Lack of Passion - Not engaging in what you love to do**
- [ ] **Stress - Job, family, finances, relationships, are just some of the stressors**
- [ ] **Other (List here)**

Common Underlying Causes Of Cravings

Dehydration – This can show up as cravings for food if you are not tapped into what you eat and drink, OR if what you eat or drink causes dehydration (sodas, diet drinks, zero calorie drinks, caffeine, energy drinks, carbonated water, fruit drinks, and so on). Dehydration is the first thing to look at when cravings arrive. Drink some purified water and see how receptive your body is to the water.

Taste/Leftovers – When you know you are full, the taste of certain foods left over in your mouth can often create cravings for more. If this happens to you, try cleaning your palette after a meal or snack. Use diluted apple cider vinegar, lemon water, brush your teeth, or use a tongue scraper.

The Void – The void is that place where you feel very alone or frustrated with a life event or reality. When you feel that void, you may turn to emotional eating, which is normal. It's important to recognize the traumas that happened to you in your early years, and how they relate to food and emotions. When there is a void, acknowledging it is a huge step towards understanding yourself and your food cravings.

Job/Career/Work – Most people spend the majority of their lives at work more than any other activity, unless you cultivate a passion. Do you love your Job/Career/Work? Are you engaging with your true passion on a daily basis? If so, great. If not – this too can create cravings to mask a sense of being unfulfilled.

Nutrient Deficient Foods – It all goes back to ingredients. If you eat a lot of processed and refined items, they deplete you of much-needed nutrients that your body tries to absorb from your food. Look at what you eat or drink, especially when you don't feel well. This will help you connect with what's really going on in your body and mood. (see Ingredientology, page 53)

Hormones – As hormones fluctuate so do your cravings. Hormone fluctuations are natural, but sometimes your hormones SCREAM out for candy, junk food, comfort foods, the drive-thru or delivery. Other times, hormones are more regulated which helps you make nourishing choices. The more you are in tune with your hormonal cycle, the more you will know how to manage your hormones. The cleaner your food, the more harmonious your hormones will become.

Seasons – Today's workforce rarely takes into consideration the seasons, and the different levels of energy you need to get through each season. As the seasons change so do your cravings and your need for certain kinds of foods. Warm weather months (spring and summer) are great for lighter, raw and refreshing foods. Winter (depending on how cold it gets where you live) is the time to hunker down and eat lots of nourishing fats, and get warming, cooked foods into your system to keep you going. Not too long ago, the autumn harvest was a time to stock up on foods for the winter so that you could slow down and also survive it. These days you can't tell what season it is by walking into the grocery store, because food comes from all over the world, instead of staying local.

Holidays – They can create HUGE obligations as well as specific food cravings. You can begin to Upgrade and enjoy the holidays once you realize what is happening with the ingredients. This is the first step towards getting you to where you want to be… awareness.

Current Events – What's happening in your life right now directly affects cravings. Do you notice how it seems more difficult to take care of yourself when someone close to you is having a crisis? Negative world events can have the same impact. Often, turning OFF the news is the best way to have a better day!

Relationships – These are a biggie. If you have loving, nurturing relationships with yourself and others, there is a sense of fulfillment. If you don't, you may experience a void and turn to drugs, alcohol, food, or 'check out' on activities such as surfing the internet or watching TV - just to make it through the day or night.

Community – Do you have the community you desire? Ancestrally, we grew up in tribes. Do you have your tribe? Do you live alone or with people you are not in alignment with? Does your home feel like a sanctuary or nurturing community? It's important to feel a sense of community – whether it's with people, pets, friends, or connecting with nature or involved in a group project.

Blood Sugar Stability – Even when you feel amazing and things are going well, if you don't pay attention to your blood sugar levels you can knock yourself out of whack. Many people skip meals and don't pay attention to the fact that they have gone too long without food. When your blood sugar drops too low, it makes your body feels as if it's in starvation mode. As a result, people impulsively go for the quickest potential 'fuel food'. It's easier to choose nourishing foods with stable blood sugar by scheduling meals and snacks. (see Blood-Sugarology page 101).

Visual Triggers – Have you noticed there are no more TV commercials about cigarettes? Why? Because we now understand how toxic cigarettes are AND how CONVINCING advertising is. It's a fact that advertising is visually stimulating and creates DESIRE. Pay attention the next time you watch TV. The majority of commercials are food manufacturers suggesting that their product is healthy. Notice how the drug commercials advertise MORE side effects than benefits. It's probable that there are fewer smokers because TV commercials for cigarettes no longer exist. Imagine what would happen if there were no more junk food or pharmaceutical commercials… something to chew on.

Your Nose! – Smells are hard to avoid. Smells can trigger cravings. Certain smells, such as coffee or freshly baked bread, get me every time. Learning to be prepared with Upgraded options can assist you and your sweet nose. Begin to carry delicious and Upgraded snacks with you to ease the temptation.

Lack of Movement – If you don't get enough movement, pent up energy can surface as agitation and using food (or other vices) is often an attempt to stuff down energy even deeper. Movement is essential, and the right movement for YOUR body type and your current ability is even more important. Starting with a small walk can do wonders and you don't have to join a gym (more on that later in Chapter 9).

Stress – All of the above are some kind of mental or physical stress on your body. Stress creates the production of cortisol. The more cortisol that is produced, the more it taxes the body (page 207).

How Cravings Connect Us To Our Past

So now that you understand what may be causing your cravings, let's look at your cravings in a different light and how they are connected to ancestry/childhood. Instead of fighting the craving, try a different approach - **HONOR your cravings**. If your grandmother gave you milk and cookies as a child before bed and you find yourself indulging in milk and cookies each night, or during a stressful event, you may not be craving the food. You may be craving the connection to a time when you felt that deep-rooted love from your grandmother. The habit is what makes you feel good, despite the chemicals in the cookies and milk that make you feel less than stellar most of the other time.

What to do about those old comforting foods?
How to handle comforting memories of certain foods & foods from your ancestry or childhood?

Recognize them: Name the comfort foods. Are they from your childhood? From your ancestry? What makes this particular food a comfort food? What is the memory associated with this food?

Upgrade: Select the healthiest possible alternative. For instance, make the most nutritious, delicious cookies and milk to honor that ritual. Just as frankenfoods will lead to inflammation and more cravings, denying yourself the ritual may lead you to binge eat those old nutrient devoid cookies and then feeling bad about it. Then you repeat the pattern over and over again. Upgrading that ritual with quality ingredients is a way to satisfy the craving AND ingest cleaner ingredients. Something to feel good about.

Upgrade Example: Use organic milk and organic (instead of refined) ingredients for your cookie. **See Upgraded Chocolate Chip Cookie recipe on page 151.**

I work with a client who grew up on a dairy farm. She knows that her body does not tolerate dairy anymore. The dairy she buys in the store is EXTREMELY different than the pure dairy she drank as a child. The ah-ha for her was to recognize her childhood lifestyle, honor it, and then find ways to keep that creamy substance in her life - without the negative side effects.

We started looking at **Upgraded ingredients** such as coconut milk, coconut butters, nut butters and nut milks to create a consistency and taste that gave her that sense of childhood comfort. Win-WIN! She is aware of the comfort foods she seeks and the related emotions tied to those foods. With that knowledge and acknowledgment, she Upgraded to ingredients that her body and mind now says ….. Ahhhhhh to. As a result, **she has satisfied her body, her fond childhood memories, her current situation AND her taste buds.**

I strongly believe you can eat whatever you want! You just need to identify what YOU really crave and WHY you crave it. Does it have to do with abundance (having too much and wanting more such as an addictive substance), or being denied something (on a diet, white knuckling, purple unicorn)? Once you know WHAT it is you want and WHY you want it, then you have the opportunity to get creative with your ingredients to make meals/snacks that satisfy and nourish **you**. With a little time and practice, Upgrading ingredients WILL become second nature.

What are the ingredients in the foods you crave & how do they affect you?

If you only get one thing out of this entire book, **READ Ingredients.** NOT the front of the box or the Nutritional Facts, but the INGREDIENTS (see page 54). This alone will educate you enough to make Upgraded choices. When you begin to really know what you put in your body, you will know what makes your body sick, moody and tired, and what makes your body feel energetic, highly functional and nourished.

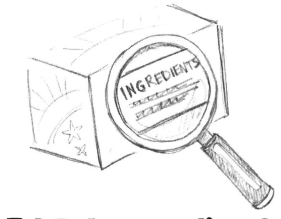

READ Ingredients

Would you put regular unleaded gasoline into a jet? Or jet fuel into a VW Bug? Why not? The proper fuel (nourishing food) will lubricate an engine (digest well) and makes it run smoothly (gives you energy). An inappropriate fuel (processed and refined frankenfoods) will gunk up the engine (your intestines) and begin to cause issues (digestive and inflammation) that turn into expensive break downs and repairs (disease).

Most people take better care of their car than they do themselves.

When a car is low on fuel, what do you do? Head for the gas station? If you've ever run out of gas (yup, I did it once) then you probably were more aware of your gas tank after that. I'm guessing it hasn't happened too many times in your driving experiences. So why do you allow your blood sugar (fuel tank) to get too low? Do you drive on empty?

Begin to read all ingredients and start to notice what you are feeling after you eat. Are you running smoothly or clunking along? Is it time to find the right fuel (nourishing food) for your engine (body)?

For instance, eating food products with MSG will CREATE cravings, disrupt your natural hunger signals, and confuse you into thinking that you are super hungry and need this other gunk food, pronto!

How can you begin to Upgrade your food? Every little thing towards eating clean and real foods counts. Just switching from the regular store version to the natural or organic version is a big Upgrade. Every little Upgrade creates that muscle you are building upon as you go through the Upgrade process.

What do you feel when you have food cravings?

Do emotions rule your world? Of course, emotions rule most of us. KNOWING that you feel angry, sad, depressed, happy, anxious, lonely, bored, restless and saying to yourself "I'm angry so I'm eating this to feel better"... can be very powerful. Honor who YOU are and what YOU feel. Us binge eaters often eat to stuff down the emotions that we don't want to feel, or our blood sugar has dropped into a danger zone.

For some reason, you received the message that you are never supposed to feel angry, tired, depressed, lonely, irritated or frustrated. Instead of fully realizing what's happening, you move away from your emotions in the form of food, drugs, alcohol, TV and so on. It's important to be aware of your true feelings and not how you think you 'should' feel. Being aware of your true feelings, without pushing them away, can be challenging for some and easy breezy for others.

Writing things down and getting them out on paper has been shown to have a powerful effect on understanding your emotions. **Try this out:**

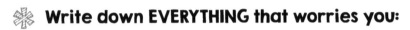 **Write down EVERYTHING that worries you:**

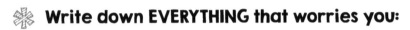 **Now go back and ~~cross off~~ anything that is out of your control.**

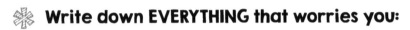 **PRIORITIZE what is left on the list and create action steps for the TOP 3:**

   1.

   2.

   3.

Craving Q's

These questions are to find out what you crave. Then begin to dig a little deeper to see how and when they come up for you. After going through some of these in detail, begin to look at Upgraded options for the items you crave.

Answer the following questions about your Cravings:

? **Do you have cravings? Yes / No**

? **If Yes, what do you crave?**

? **When do you crave?** Time of day? Specific Places? Certain Emotions?

? **How do you know you are satisfied after you've had a craving?**

? **What are the ways that have worked for you to curb a craving?**

? **Based on the above, what is one new way that you can approach your cravings?**

Example: I notice that when I don't eat breakfast, I tend to eat more and more as the evening goes on. I usually end up with an overstuffed belly at bedtime. When I eat breakfast in the morning and have snacks every few hours, then I don't tend to binge in the evening. When I nourish myself during the day, I notice I'm more satisfied just to drink liquids in the evening after dinner (instead of munching on food all night).

You **CAN** understand your food cravings. It requires some planning and thinking ahead. By staying hydrated and Upgrading trigger foods, you can tame the cravings beast. When cravings happen, it's essential to have healthy options available and keep in mind the benefits of selecting nourishing foods versus the consequences of choosing harmful trigger foods. Keep snacks with you so that you don't get to a point of feeling extremely hungry. When cravings occur, it's not about testing your willpower but understanding and satisfying your craving with healthful and nourishing Upgrades/alternatives.

Upgrade Your Cravings

The Importance of Breakfast & Being Prepared With Snacks

Why is breakfast considered the most important meal of the day? It's essential that you **eat a nourishing breakfast** to kick off your morning **with blood sugar stabilization.** Also, don't forget to snack on healthy foods throughout your day. Without a fuel-filled breakfast and snacks, your blood sugar will probably drop and you may get really hungry. As a result, you give into unhealthy food cravings because they are so convenient and will **appear** as instant fuel. **See Breakfast & Snacks,** in Chapter 5 (page 112-114) for more tips!

Fast Carbs vs Slow Carbs

The types of carbs you eat also help you avoid binge eating on foods that don't nourish your body. So what carbs could you eat and what could you Upgrade? Upgrade the fast carbs (simple carbohydrates). Fast carbs include processed breads, refined sugars, etc. Slow carbs, also known as complex carbohydrates, are the Upgraded choice and give you more energy throughout your day. Slow carbs are mostly vegetables, legumes, whole grains, etc. **See Fast Carbs, Fruit Carbs & Slow Carbs** in Chapter 5 (page 116).

What Food Does Your Body REALLY Crave?

Often when you crave a certain food, you really lack specific minerals in your body and you are actually craving that nutrient (and not the artificial, processed food you THINK you need). It can be difficult to think about nutrients in the middle of a craving, so it's important to be aware before cravings hit. I find that some of the biggest cravings stem from the following:

1. Lack of nourishing foods and dehydration.
2. Blood sugar dropping too low/ going too long without food.
3. Eating foods that are highly processed and aggravate your energy, emotions, and rationale.

	For example, if you crave:
Sugar	You may be deficient in chromium, carbon, phosphorus, etc. Think about having organic veggies, fruits, and/or a handful of nuts or seeds with you.
Salt	You may be deficient in chloride and silicon. Instead, plan ahead to eat nuts and seeds. Cashews, chia seeds, pumpkin seeds are all excellent choices.
Fast Carbs (bread, pasta etc.)	You may be deficient in nitrogen. Plan ahead and stock up on protein-rich foods such as organic beans, asparagus or chia seeds for Vegans. Grass-fed/Grass-finished meat and/or wild-caught fatty fish for meat eaters.
Fried/Oily Foods	You may be deficient in calcium. Have on hand green leafy veggies or avocados.

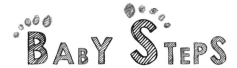

 **Write down a food/drink that you often crave:**

 **What are the ingredients of this food/drink?** Yup, write down ALL of the ingredients:

 **Go to recipe/ingredient conversion** in Chapter 6, page 151-156 (if you don't already have a recipe) and alter the recipe using Upgraded ingredients so it's both delicious and satisfying to you.

Write your Upgraded recipe here:

Now that you understand your cravings and why it's important to honor them, let's dive into one of the most important and sometimes hard to recognize signs… **dehydration**.

WATER

I was shocked to find out that a friend recently turned 55. Honestly, I thought she was in her late 30's. We talked about her youthful looks at her 55th birthday party and she spilled the beans. Her secret is… Water! She said that when she was a little girl she found out just how much our bodies are made of water. Since her looks were very important to her, she decided then that she would always drink about half her body weight in ounces of water each day. She jokes about how much she goes to the bathroom, but says it's well worth it given how beautiful and nearly wrinkle-free her youthful 55 year-old skin looks.

Forget that gimmicky anti-wrinkle cream and the plastic, chemical products people want to sell you for beautiful skin! Instead, invest in the best water filter you can. In the long run, this will be much cheaper than buying useless (and often toxic-riddled) products. You know that water is good for you, but sometimes it feels difficult or boring to drink, especially when surrounded by much sexier-looking and tasting drinks.

Percentage of water in the body
* 70-75% of the body is WATER
* 75% of muscle is WATER
* 90% of the brain is WATER
* 22% of bones are WATER
* 83% of blood is WATER

That's a lot of water! As a result, it's important to replenish that water in order to stay hydrated, lubricated, and functioning optimally.

Purified Water helps you in the following ways:
* Assists nutrients and oxygen into the blood cells
* Assists a well-functioning metabolism
* Regulates body temperature
* Keeps the air in lungs moist
* Keeps joints lubricated
* Assists with necessary detoxification
* Releases the pain of headaches or migraines (dehydration)
* Aids in weight loss
* Creates healthier looking and feeling skin
* Assists in clearer thinking
* Increases energy
* Assists with digestion when drinking 20 minutes before a meal
* Relieves constipation
* Reduces cramping
* Is an overall feel-good pick-me-up!

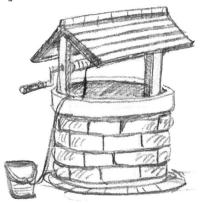

Some signs that you may be dehydrated

☐ **Dry skin**

☐ **Dry Mouth**

☐ **Headache**

☐ **Dizziness or Lightheadedness**

☐ **Dark and/or strong smelling urine.** Urine should be pale yellow or clear.

☐ **Thirst** - if you get to the point where you feel thirsty, you are already dehydrated. Drinking room temperature purified water at this point will help to hydrate you more than drinking cold water.

☐ **Fatigue** - if you feel unnecessarily tired, check your water intake and increase. Drinking enough water will help increase energy and make you feel better.

☐ **Hunger close to after eating a meal** - especially after eating processed, refined, or water-devoid foods.

The hunger (via dehydration) thing perplexed me for quite a long time until I started drinking enough water and to my delight found that I did not have as many cravings. It also did wonders for my skin. I moved to the high desert and noticed some people with very dry skin. My skin then started to dry out but once I really nourished myself with enough water, I then dispelled the myth that living in the desert dries out your skin.

It's important to know which symptoms you have so that you can measure your progress.

? **Do you have any of the signs of dehydration? If so, which ones?**

? **Are you convinced you need to drink lots of purified water? Yes / No**

? **How much are you currently drinking?**

Drink Purified Water
Get a filtration system that fits your budget!

The best water is freshly filtered water. Water that sits in plastic bottles for a prolonged period of time, especially in heat, releases toxins from the plastic and into the water. The least expensive way to get purified water is to buy a faucet filter system, or to find a purified water system (located at most health food stores or search and purchase online) and purchase it/refill bottles by the gallon.

Most tap water is full of chlorine and fluoride. Fluoride may contain:

* Lead
* Cadmium
* Mercury
* Arsenic

Fluoride may also contribute to the following health problems:

* Neurological/brain issues
* Kidney problems
* Chronic fatigue
* Gastrointestinal
* Hyperactivity
* Immune system issues

Yikes. Not convinced? As always, do the research for yourself. I, for one, get a stomachache EVERY single time I have tap water. I'm not a fan of purchasing single bottles of water. Instead, I choose to buy my water from a health food store water purifying machine. Fill up your own bottles and go from there. You can research to find out about the water quality in your area. The research I've done shows that fluoride can be quite toxic. Conduct your own research and decide what is best for you and your family.

Slowly increase the amount of water you drink!

You can do this by drinking water first thing in the morning. Start with 6-12 ounces first thing in the morning and before each meal or snack. Make it a habit to always have water with you to sip throughout the day. Preferably, your water container is glass or metal or at least BPA-free plastic. NEVER leave a plastic water bottle in a hot car or anywhere hot because chemicals from the plastic can leach into your drinking water.

Caffeine, sugar drinks, artificial flavor drinks, etc. do NOT count as water.

These popular beverages dehydrate you MORE and create MORE cravings because you don't realize you are dehydrated. See Upgraded Beverages (page 142) to discover your new hydrating beverage.

Dehydrating:

Coffee of any kind, caffeinated teas, energy drinks (surprise), most sports drinks, excess carbonated water, soda/diet soda (of any kind), etc.

Hydrating:

Lemon or Lime water, Organic Raw Apple Cider Vinegar diluted in water, Coconut water (from a pure source, not from concentrate), Chia water, and regular purified water.

YES, natural herbal teas are fine for your water consumption. Make sure the water tastes naturally good to you. You can also add in Chia seeds to water to assist in better hydration with less water. Add Organic RAW Apple Cider Vinegar, lemon, or slices of fruit or berries for flavor and nutrients.

If your goal is 100 ounces of Purified water per day:

Day 1 – 10 oz	Day 6 – 35 oz	Day 11 – 60 oz	Day 17 – 85 oz
Day 2 – 15 oz	Day 7 – 40 oz	Day 12 – 65 oz	Day 18 – 90 oz
Day 3 – 20 oz	Day 8 – 45 oz	Day 13 – 70 oz	Day 19 – 95 oz
Day 4 – 25 oz	Day 9 – 50 oz	Day 14 – 75 oz	Day 20 – 100 oz
Day 5 – 30 oz	Day 10 – 55 oz	Day 15 – 80 oz	Day 21 – 100 oz

Quicker you say? Increase by 8 ounces per day:

Day 1 – 18 oz	Day 4 – 42 oz	Day 7 – 66 oz	Day 10 – 90 oz
Day 2 – 26 oz	Day 5 – 50 oz	Day 8 – 74 oz	Day 11 – 98 oz
Day 3 – 34 oz	Day 6 – 58 oz	Day 9 – 82 oz	Day 12 – 100 oz

Helpful Water Tips

* **Hydrate in the morning:** Pour 8-20 oz of warm or room temperature purified water, and squeeze one-half of a **lemon** into water. Drink or sip, and then wait at least 20 minutes before eating breakfast. You can also drink it 20 minutes before each meal and it's a great pre-workout energy drink. Ideally, use organic lemons and freshly squeeze them yourself. You can make a few days' worth of lemon water at a time and store in the fridge.

Lemon Benefits:
  * Antiviral, antibacterial, and immune boosting.
  * Natural breath freshener and helps keep you hydrated.
  * Contains enzymes which stimulate detoxification from the liver.
  * Enhances weight release, is a digestive aide and a natural cravings buster.
  * Helps to flush out your system of toxins and helps strengthen urinary tract.
  * Increases energy and the smell of lemon can help clear your mind and enhance your mood.
  * Contains magnesium, Vitamin C, calcium, and bioflavonoids that increase immunity.

* My favorite is to drink 12-20 oz of warm water with 1 TBSP Organic Raw **Apple Cider Vinegar** first thing in the morning. I will also create a 32 ounce container of this drink to go and drink 8-10 ounces (20 minutes before each meal). This drink hydrates and kick starts the digestive system. Many people have found healing with just the Organic RAW Apple Cider Vinegar drinks alone. Make sure it's RAW, Organic and Unfiltered! *Always dilute Apple Cider Vinegar. Page 31.

* A client wanted to be sure to get in 64 oz of water each day. She got four 16 oz glass bottles and filled them up in the morning. She set them on the counter, drank one before leaving for work, took the other two with her to work, and then had one more when she got home from work. This helped her keep track of the water she wanted to drink without carrying around a 64 oz jug.

Explore to see what works for YOU and your daily water intake!

Recommendation

Use Glass or Stainless steel bottles. One of the benefits of using glass is that it won't leach chemicals. I especially recommend this if you live in a hot climate as heat creates the leaching of toxins from plastic. You can order online 16, 24 or 32-ounce ball jars that are very inexpensive and are a great way to keep track of how much water you drink on a daily basis. Most plastics contain BPA, which is a chemical that may have harmful health effects. There are BPA-free bottles available (use these only in mild climate). If you drink from plastic, the bottles should never be microwaved or left inside a hot place or car.

WATER Questions

How much water do you think you drink?_____

Calculate the optimal amount of water for **YOU**:
How much do you weigh _____
Divide by 1/2 _____
(This is the total number of **OUNCES** of water to move towards drinking per day)
Take at least 10 days of slowly increasing to get to your desired amount of water.

Why do I recommend slowly increasing your water? (*Image: Toilet paper dragging behind on shoe*) Unless you love going to the bathroom ALL the time, increasing your water too much (and too quickly) may lead to a deterrent. It's annoying to constantly run to the bathroom all day. If you spread out the water and sip throughout the day, then you are nourished, hydrated and you aren't glued to the porcelain.

Here are more questions to consider!

? **What kind of filtration works for me and my budget today?**

? **What kind of filtration system would I like in the future?**

? **When will I purchase it?**

? **How many days do I want to take to increase my water from _____ oz (current amount) to (YOUR optimal amount) _____oz?**

? **How does this plan feel to me?**

? **Why do I need more water?**

? **What do I hope it will do for me?**

? **When will I begin to drink more water? (Hint: Today's a Good Day for that!)**

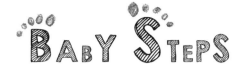

 Determine how much water you are currently drinking and increase by 10-12 oz today: What is that amount_____

 Begin to drink 6-8 oz of water 20 minutes before breakfast. Once that feels comfortable, add in another 6-8 oz before lunch and then dinner:

 Determine approximately half your body weight in ounces: _____
For Example: 200lbs = 100 oz. Half of that amount = 50 oz.
Slowly increase by a few ounces a day until you reach your optimal amount of daily water: Then re-assess: Is this too much water for you? **Or not enough?** Check the list on page 47 to see if you experience any symptoms related to dehydration.

I highly recommend re-visiting this chapter from time to time. Cravings can be tricky! The more you are aware of how your cravings contribute to a multitude of physical and emotional imbalances, the closer you are to finding the pieces that solves your cravings puzzle.

In Chapter 2 we discussed:

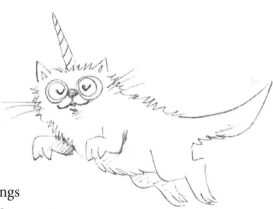

* Willpower
* Famous Failures
* The importance of honoring your cravings
* Understanding cravings from their roots
* The Purple Unicorn
* Patterns and possibilities for cravings
* All calories are NOT created equal
* Getting curious about the ingredients you crave
* Being aware of what and when you have specific carvings
* How to begin thinking about Upgrading your cravings
* The importance of hydration

We explored why it's important to understand the messages and meanings that linger around your cravings. You also learned that honoring and recognizing your food cravings are far more important than trying to deny them.

In Chapter 3, you will learn about the #1 thing you need in order to Upgrade your Food and Upgrade your Life. **INGREDIENTS!** You will learn how to truly read and understand ingredients in a way that you may have overlooked all this time. **So many people 'think' they eat healthy** yet they are being deceived by marketing and packaging. Learn what's really inside your food!

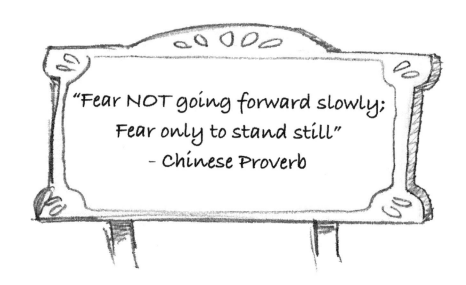

"Fear NOT going forward slowly;
Fear only to stand still"
- Chinese Proverb

3 INGREDIENTOLOGY

The Importance of Reading Ingredients
(Not Nutritional Facts)

Ingredientology is simple:

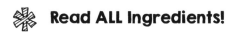 **Read ALL Ingredients!**

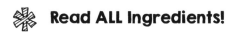 **Begin to understand what the ingredients are!**

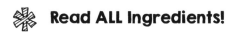 **Make it a ritual to always read ingredients! EVEN IF you purchased the product before.**

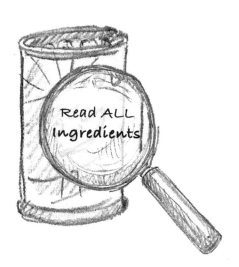

Read ALL Ingredients

Ingredients can change without noticing a difference in the packaging.

Marketers and advertisers will promote any benefits they can muster and leave out the undesirables. Advertising is a multi-billion dollar industry and they are paid the big bucks to be convincing. They can call a product 'all natural' and it can be filled with chemicals. They can call a product 'fiber and protein rich' and it can be filled with MSG, refined sugar and GMO's. They can call a product 'organic' with the organic ingredients being minimal and overpowered by chemicals.

Don't Judge a Product by its Nutritional Facts

Forgeddabout it! Don't worry about what the nutritional label says either. A nutritious looking product can call itself all-natural, fiber and vitamin packed, and still be loaded with chemicals. You don't know what's really going on with your food until you read the… **I N G R E D I E N T S**. Otherwise, you are buying a mystery package because you *think* it's going to have something lucky inside it.

Bottom Line: Don't believe the Packaging a.k.a. Marketing. Would you buy a used car (without looking under the hood or test driving it) from a stranger you accidentally met in a parking lot?

If you only get one thing out of this entire book, Read Ingredients!

Repeat: If you only get ONE thing out of this entire book, Read ALL Ingredients.

And just to drive it home, if you only do just ONE thing (sing along)
READ ALL INGREDIENTS…Always!

If you understand the ingredients, then you are closer to understanding what you really put into your body. And those mysterious ailments might not be so confusing anymore.

If the INGREDIENTS are good, then the product is good!

If the INGREDIENTS are toxic, then the product is TOXIC!

Simple as that!

Many people **think** they eat healthy until they start to **read** and **understand** ingredients. I've had more clients than I can count come to me and say that they eat extremely healthy. However, they work with me because they have a multitude of undesirable symptoms but reassure me that it's not THEIR food (and some of these folks are very convincing)! Because they don't think it's their food, they don't write in the Food/Mood Journal that I recommend. I'll ask them about their eating habits, and they even tell me they eat organic food and read ingredients. However, every time they do their Food/Mood Journal and begin to read and report back the true ingredients in their food, they are terribly surprised at what they find.

You may THINK you know how to read ingredients, but you may just be looking at the nutritional facts. The advertising on the front of the box/package may **convince** you that the food is 'healthy'.

When you start to truly read ingredients (NOT nutritional facts) and notice how your food affects you, you probably will be shocked, surprised and dismayed at what you find in your food. When my clients start to Upgrade, they are pleasantly surprised at how much better they feel (increased energy, decreased symptoms) and how much they still enjoy their food. A client said it well, *"If I don't understand the ingredients, I put the package down and if I want it bad enough, I'll look up the mysterious ingredients."*

In the end, this is a great feeling for both me and my clients. They know what is in their food and the ailments that may be associated with these foods. It makes me feel really great about educating my clients and contributing to their health and healing. I love to help people feel better!

If you think your food is stellar and that your symptoms can't possibly result from the food you eat, I challenge you to **become an INGREDIENTOLOGIST**.

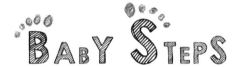

Read EVERY INGREDIENT and begin to UNDERSTAND what is TRULY inside YOUR FOOD!

BaBy Steps

Read the ingredients of foods in your home. Did you find any surprising ingredients? If so, write them here:

Begin to read the ingredients while shopping in the grocery store. Any surprises? NOTE them here:

Begin to ask for the ingredients in restaurants or places you go to eat. Any surprises? Write them here:

Organics

Before chemical farming, all foods were "organic". Organic means that foods were grown and prepared without chemical fertilizers, pesticides, herbicides, and irradiation. In the good ol' days foods were grown and harvested in harmony with nature. With chemical farming and food production moving into factories, heavy processing has depleted nutrients in foods.

The process of 'mono-cropping' (planting the same crop repeatedly such as soy, wheat, corn, etc.) also depletes the soil of nutrients; whereas, nature's cycle is far more organic and nutritious.

If you have ever visited an organic backyard farm, you know what I'm talking about. Plants that grow together create harmony and if planted thoughtfully, many plants will act as natural bug deterrents. For example, mint deters ants from entering your garden. Lavender deter fleas, and basil can discourage mosquitoes.

Pesticides do more harm than good and it's easy to become extremely toxic when continually exposed to these chemicals.

Pesticides have been linked with the following:

* Cancer
* Infertility
* Nausea
* Vomiting
* Diarrhea
* Allergies
* Asthma
* Neurological issues
* Liver, kidney & blood diseases
* Weakened immune system
* Skin issues such as rashes
* ADD
* ADHD
* Birth defects

Organics & Future Generations

Organics help protect our future and environment. The more we invest in organic farmers, the more we invest in natural, nutrient-rich soil and clean foods for generations to come. Organics help our water supply; where do you think the run-off from sprayed chemicals goes? They flow into our rivers, oceans, and other water sources. When crop planes dust the crops, these pesticides are carried through the air to crops, neighboring farms, to unsuspecting people and their homes.

Organics help sustain our precious farmers. Most organic farms are tiny compared to the mass mono-cropped and chemically-driven farms. We need to support them so that we can continue to access clean, organic foods. This also creates a true economy where money goes into much deserved small and family farms. If we don't support the small organic farmers they will be bought out by the corporations and turned into more chemical farming.

Organics Shopping Tips
Why Buy Organic?

Organics taste so much better. Do a comparison yourself. Buy a conventional (GMO) fruit or vegetable from the supermarket and then buy an organic version from your local co-op, natural grocery store, farm, or Farmer's Market. Taste each one and then compare. I'm sure you can definitely tell the difference between the GMO vs. NON-GMO produce. Weigh the options for yourself.

Yes, organics can sometimes be a jump in price. If you find yourself saying that Organics are too expensive… please answer the following questions. These questions will help you realize that organics are CHEAPER in the long run.

- **?** How much do you spend on medical issues each month?
- **?** Medications?
- **?** Are you lethargic, have gut issues, headaches, allergies or brain fog?
- **?** Are you missing out on activities you enjoy because you don't have the energy or feel well?

Processed and Fast Foods Can Lead to Huge Medical Expenses!

Isn't it worth paying a little more in order to feel healthier and lead a more fulfilled life? A great way to save money on organics is to buy in season. Join a CSA (Community Supported Agriculture http://www.localharvest.org/csa/) if there is one located in your area. Another option is to visit natural food markets and ask where they keep the foods that can no longer be displayed. Stores won't display fruits and veggies that are beyond prime. Did you know that you are better off eating wilted organic produce than eating conventional ones that look good? If you have room, consider starting a small garden or grow your own sprouts (see Chapter 8, page 184 on How to Grow Your Own Sprouts).

While fresh is best, the next alternative is organic frozen food. When you find organic frozen food items on sale that you enjoy, stock up. To save money, look for organics that are in season and/or purchase produce that is on sale. Ask your local organic grocer to save the 'throw-way' produce for you.

Money-Saving Tips

* Search online for organic coupons and promotions (most stores will also accept competitor coupons).
* **See Shopping Guide on page 187 for more ideas!**

As you begin your transition to organics, you **WILL** taste and feel the difference. You will also make a significant contribution to the hard working organic farmers, to your health and to the health of future generations. With Organics you *"Put your money where your mouth is!"*

How to Understand Produce Labels & Stickers

When you buy fruits and vegetables from the market, pay attention to labels and stickers. These stickers are called the **PLU** (Price Look Up) code. The last four numbers on the code explain which fruit or vegetable it is. For example, the last four digits on a small Fuji apple are 4131, bananas are 4011, and Meyer lemons are 3626, etc.

If the PLU sticker has only **FOUR numbers**, then the produce **was exposed to pesticides**. This is sometimes called traditional or conventional methods. Sad but true. If a small Fuji apple has a 4131 PLU sticker (four numbers only) then it was grown using pesticides/herbicides.

If the PLU sticker has **FIVE numbers** in the code starting with an **"8"**, then it's a **Genetically Modified Organism (GMO)** fruit or vegetable. A GMO banana would be 84011.

If the PLU sticker has **FIVE numbers** in the PLU code starting with a **"9"**, then it was grown with **organic standards**. An organic banana would be 94011.

Recap

4011 4 Numbers = **Grown with pesticides/herbicides**

84011 5 Numbers beginning with "8" = **GMO**

 94011 5 Numbers beginning with "9" = **Organic**

If you want to educate yourself further and stay up-to-date with PLU codes, I recommend the following website: www.ewg.org/foodnews. **These are some of the MOST important items to purchase organic.** The conventional or non-organic versions of these crops are some of the most heavily sprayed and manipulated crops.

* Strawberries
* Celery
* Apples
* Peaches

* Nectarines
* Lettuce
* Blueberries
* All Leafy Greens

* Cucumbers
* Potatoes
* Cucumbers
* All peppers

* Grapes
* Corn
* Wheat
* Soy

If you cannot purchase organics, these fruits and vegetables are said to absorb fewer pesticides than others. This is either due to their tough outer skin or because of how they are traditionally grown. **If you have any serious medical issues, I recommend sticking with organics.**

* Grapefruit
* Pineapples
* Avocado

* Mushrooms
* Cantaloupe
* Sweet potatoes

* Eggplant
* Kiwi
* Watermelon

* Mangoes
* Onions
* Cabbage

Nourishing Foods

What are nourishing foods? Nourishing foods are delicious to you, healing, have vitamins, minerals and nutrients in them naturally. They are not chemically altered and remain close to their natural state. Some foods (i.e. raw sauerkraut, kefir, etc.) are fermented in a natural way to enhance the nutrients of the food or combined ingredients.

Nourishing Fats and Oils

Benefits:

* When fats are part of your meal, they create slower nutrient absorption which makes you feel FULLER longer, a good thing!
* Nourishing fats deliver fat-soluble vitamins such as A, D, E & K
* Assist with mineral absorption
* Beneficial to beautiful skin
* Excellent brain food

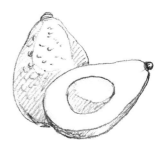

Plant-Based:

* Organic Extra Virgin Coconut Oil (many uses - can be used raw and remains stable at high heat)
* Organic Extra Virgin Olive Oil (not for cooking, best to drizzle on food after it's cooked)
* Avocado
* Nuts/Seeds
* Chia Seeds
* Ground Flax Seeds

Animal-Based:

* Organic Grass Fed/Grass Finished Butter
* Organic Grass Fed/Grass Finished Ghee (clarified butter) - also good for high heat if you don't like coconut oil
* Organic Grass Fed/Pasture Raised Animal Fat
* Yolks of Organic Pasture Raised Eggs

Organic Raw Olives and Organic Extra Virgin Olive Oil:

* Can assist with blood sugar stabilization.
* Olive Oil is a mono-unsaturated fat so it's the good fat. Be sure to find a quality olive oil. Many generic brands are cut with other toxic oils such as canola and other vegetable oils.

Organic Butter

* Real butter (from an organic source) is loaded with minerals and vitamins including: selenium (an antioxidant), A, D, E, and K2.
* Good quality fatty acids that enhance the immune system, boost metabolism, and are anti-microbial.

* Always try to get organic, but even regular butter is BETTER than margarine or ANY of the fake stuff. The less it's processed, the more it has its nutrients intact.
* Organic Ghee (Clarified butter) Many people who are dairy intolerant have found that they can eat Ghee. Ghee is made by simmering raw milk which usually removes the casein and lactose (casein and lactose are usually the irritant associated with dairy intolerance, also known as lactose-intolerant). The best Ghee will lab test their product to make sure it is gluten and casein- free.
* Pasture-raised animal fat (lard, duck fat, suet, etc.) In the old days, people cooked with lard, suet, and duck fat. If you can get clean sources and are not opposed to using them, they are filled with nutrients and are stable at high heat.

Margarine WARNING! Margarine is HIGHLY Processed. Usually Full of FAKE Ingredients including hydrogenated oils, artificial ingredients and food coloring... just to begin with.

Cholesterol and its bad rap

Beneficial cholesterol from quality fats and oils promotes a healthy brain and nervous system. Negative cholesterol issues arise from toxic fats and oils, NOT the clean and nourishing ones listed on the previous page. If you worry about your cholesterol, stick with the plant-based fats mentioned, as they do not have any cholesterol. That's right, coconut oil has ZERO cholesterol. Avocados, nuts, and seeds have ZERO cholesterol. I urge you to educate yourself more about cholesterol. A great source is the book: Nourishing Traditions by Sally Fallon.

Mineral Rich Salts

Table salt is completely devoid of nutrients. However, Himalayan Salt and Celtic Sea Salt are FULL of nutrients and minerals. They also bring out the natural flavors which makes food taste great. If your Upgraded food tastes delicious, you are more likely to stay satisfied with it.

Leafy Vegetables

There are many different types of green vegetables that you can incorporate into your meals and the nutritional benefits are huge! Even if you only get one leafy green vegetable onto your plate, it's better than none! They are high in calcium, iron, potassium, magnesium, and Vitamins A, C, E, and K. All of these nutrients are important for your body's overall health. I urge you to eat organic vegetables whenever possible. Including leafy green veggies into your food plan will increase energy and may help prevent and relieve chronic illness.

There are many different types of leafy green vegetables available! Here are just a few.

* Romaine
* Green leaf lettuce
* Bok Choy
* Kale
* Mustard greens
* Arugula
* Spinach
* Cabbage - (especially RAW Sauerkraut)
* Beet greens
* Swiss Chard

Leafy Greens

Many people get into a rut when eating raw leafy greens so mix it up and cook them sometimes. Steam, boil, sauté in water or nourishing fats, or make a salad with them. When cooking greens, boil them less than one minute to retain nutrients. Boiling has another benefit too: the green tinted water is full of nutrients that can be added to broth or tea.

Onion Family

Vegetables from the onion family add a lot of flavor to your foods!

* Onions
* Garlic
* Chives
* Scallions
* Shallots
* Leeks

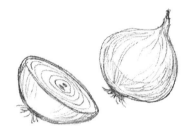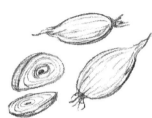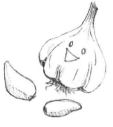

Benefits

* Controls blood sugar spikes and lowers blood sugar levels
* Prevents stroke and heart disease due to diabetes
* Packed full of Vitamin C
* Loaded with phytonutrients and dietary fiber
* Garlic: balances blood sugar, helps the pancreas function, and is a powerful anti-parasitic

Grapefruit

Grapefruit is low on the glycemic index (a system that ranks foods on a scale from 1-100 based on how certain foods affect blood sugar levels). Grapefruit also has an abundance of antioxidants such as Vitamin C and lycopene which boosts immunity and prevents cell damage. It's rich in pectin, an enzyme that helps control blood sugar. Grapefruit is rich in flavonoids and helps the liver burn surplus fats instead of allowing them to accumulate in the body.

* If you are on ANY MEDICATIONS. Ask Your Doctor first before eating grapefruit!

Eat and juice the real fruit! Fruit juices made from concentrate have been flash pasteurized which destroys the nutrients and digestive enzymes. With most bottled fruit juices, you are getting mostly fructose (refined sugar). Juice the real fruit, or even better – EAT the real fruit. There are some 'cold press' organic juices in the market today. These do not go through the pasteurization process and are an excellent Upgrade. Remember to Read Ingredients. **See Magic Trio Combinations on page 101 for more Blood Sugar Stabilizing Tips!**

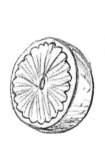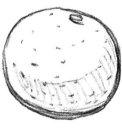

Whole Grains

A grain is considered whole when it contains all of its original parts and nutrients. Whole grains are high in fiber and require low levels of insulin to digest. White flour and white rice have been refined or milled which removes essential nutrients and converts them into sugar. Without the essential nutrients intact the white grains turn into sugar. It moves from a slow carb to a fast carb because it has been processed and is no longer a whole grain. Fast carbs create quick blood sugar spikes and drops. Slow carbs can balance and sustain blood sugar levels.

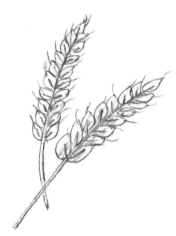

Glutenous Whole Grains

* Wheat
* Kamut
* Rye
* Spelt
* Barley

Gluten-FREE Whole Grains

* Buckwheat
* Sorghum
* Amaranth
* Teff
* Millet
* Brown & Basmati Rice
* Gluten-Free Oats

Beans/Legumes

Beans are packed with fiber and can assist with weight loss and blood sugar regulation.

* Lentils
* Black Beans
* Navy Beans
* Adzuki Beans
* Chickpeas (Garbanzo)
* Pinto Beans
* Kidney Beans
* Lima Beans
* Mung Beans
* Split Peas

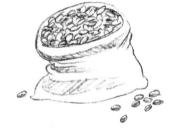

Nuts and Seeds

* Excellent nutrient dense food.

* Nuts and seeds are rich in healthy mono-unsaturated fats, antioxidants, vitamins, and minerals. They are high in protein, have a very low glycemic index, and promote cardiovascular health.

* Almonds, Walnuts, Pumpkin Seeds, Sesame Seeds and Sunflower Seeds are beneficial because they are high in protein, magnesium, and many essential nutrients. They are low on the glycemic index which helps stabilize your blood sugar.

* Brazil Nuts are high in selenium, an essential nutrient known to have anti-cancer benefits.

* Cashews, Chestnuts, Hazelnuts, Macadamia, Pecans, Pine Nuts, and Pistachios are high in potassium which protect the heart and brain.

* Flax Seeds are part of your fiber, protein and fat combination (see Magic Trio Combination on page 101) for blood sugar stabilization. They are also a great source of magnesium and potassium. They can be used as egg replacer and a natural thickening agent.

Peanut Caution:
Upgrade peanuts! Make sure they are Organic & Non-Hydrogenated.

Peanuts are most susceptible to fungus and mold. If you do eat them, buy them fresh and store them in the refrigerator because they go rancid quickly. I recommend Upgrading to Almonds!

All nuts and nut butters should be stored in the refrigerator. If you purchase nuts and seeds from the bulk bins, make sure to ask if they are emptied and cleaned frequently. If they are not cleaned frequently, then most of them could be rancid. Stick to organic, raw or dry roasted and salt-free and then add your own Celtic Sea Salt. Most people don't like the taste of nuts and seeds without salt, but add your own because table salt has anti-caking chemicals and dextrose (which is sugar derived from GMO corn).

Enjoy nuts and seeds in combination with other foods. Nut butters are also delicious. Find nut butters that do not include other ingredients in them. Mix them with vegetables so that the fiber in the vegetables can aid digestion. See Magic Trio Combinations on page 101.

Essential Omega-3 Fatty Acids

If you eat fish, make sure it is wild-caught and fresh. **'Farmed' fish are in a similar category of 'Factory Farmed' animals.** Taking them out of their natural element, into a small enclosed area for the main purpose of ease and profit. Farmed Fish and Factory Farmed animals create dis-harmony and disease within the animals and those who consume them. Omega-3s contain eicosapentaenoic acid (EPA) which stimulates the secretion of a hormone (leptin) that helps regulate food intake, body weight, and metabolism. Omega-3s help reduce inflammation. Chronic low-grade inflammation is linked to both insulin resistance and high levels of glucose.

Great Sources of Omega-3s:

* Purslane
* Hemp Seeds
* Brussels Sprouts
* Chia Seeds
* Flax Seeds
* Wild Caught Fish

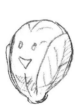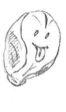

Nourishing Protein

If you are a meat eater, grass-fed/grass-finished or green-fed meats are a must. Just search the internet for factory farming, and you too will convert to pasture raised, grass fed, hormone and antibiotic-free meat and poultry. The hormones and antibiotics given to factory farmed animals create dis-harmony in YOUR system. You do not know what you are ingesting when you eat these toxic meats and dairy products. As mentioned in the Organics section, GO ORGANIC! You and your health are worth every penny! Organics will keep you healthier, and save you an extraordinary amount of money, time, and effort in the long run.

Clean Sources:

* Grass Fed, Grass Finished or Green Fed Meat
* Wild Caught - Sustainable Fish
* Pasture Raised, Free Range, Antibiotic/Hormone Free Poultry and Eggs
* Their **feed** (food) should also be **NON-GMO** and ideally **Soy-Free**

Probiotic Foods

Some healing probiotics are lactobacillus and bifid bacterium. If you eat dairy, then find an organic yogurt or kefir. My favorite probiotic food is RAW Sauerkraut. Probiotic foods increase the GOOD gut flora, and aid in digestion and absorption of nutrients. Probiotics are also an essential role in the body's immune defenses. If you don't eat probiotic foods, then I recommend to experiment with them or find a high-quality probiotic supplement. See Probiotic Foods on page 122 for more details.

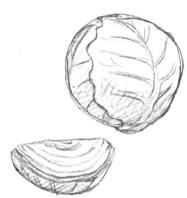

Flavor

It's all about flavor-enhancing sauces that make your food taste delicious! See sauce and dressing recipes for more inspiration (See "It's All About The Sauce" on page 106).

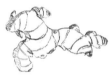

Organic Spices

* Such as turmeric, cinnamon, fenugreek, cilantro, coriander, chili pepper, and ginger. Turmeric is an amazing anti-inflammatory! Ceylon Cinnamon can help regulate blood sugar.
* Curry – is a blend of spices that often includes: turmeric, cinnamon, cilantro, coriander, chili peppers, and ginger.

Allergy Warning:

If you have a known allergy to any of these foods and want to try an alternative, test out an Upgraded version. If you desire something you are allergic to (such as gluten), look for the cleanest Upgrades and get creative.

Fill Up Faster and Stay Satisfied with Healing Foods

Foods that have a higher calorie to weight ratio tend to fill you up faster. Foods that contain large amounts of harmful fats, sugars and chemicals (i.e. white bread, pastries, fast food, MSG-laden and processed snack foods) tend to leave you wanting more and more and more! Find Upgraded foods that satisfy you and fill you up.

Foods that contain a large amount of water, dietary fiber and/or protein like fruit and nuts have the highest fullness factor. Think about Fiber, Fat, and Protein (Magic Trio Combination, page 101) at each meal or snack. By eating more healing foods, you will feel fuller and more satisfied with your food. It can help cut out the cravings for the processed and refined foods as well. 100 calories of vegetables are not the same as 100 calories from processed/refined foods. I encourage you to stop counting calories and start READING and understanding ingredients. **All calories are NOT the same!** See Chapter 7 starting on page 161 for more Healing Foods.

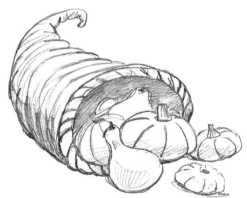

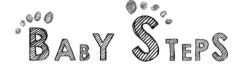

BaBy StepS

Go through this chapter and highlight items you would like to incorporate as Upgrades:

Write down a few items that looked interesting to you that you would enjoy trying:

Read Ingredients, Investigate Ingredients & Begin to Understand the INGREDIENTS in the foods YOU tend towards:

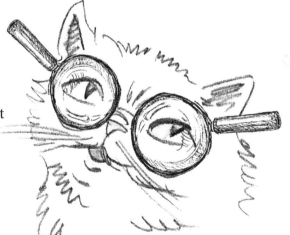

In Chapter 3, we discussed:

* The importance of becoming an Ingredientologist
* Don't judge a product by it's nutritional label
* The importance of Organics
* How to understand PLU codes
* Intro to Nourishing Foods
* Clean sources of Omega 3's and Protein
* The benefits of Probiotic Foods
* How to fill up and stay satisfied with healing foods

In Chapter 4, we'll take this exploration of ingredients another step further. You'll learn about the harmful effects of refined sugar and artificial sweeteners (i.e. found in sodas and refined, chemically-processed frankenfoods). You'll learn how to slowly detox from sugar, and how to still honor your SWEET cravings with more nourishing and Upgraded sweeteners.

He approaches me so smooth

With succulent promises

Of taste and texture

His aroma draws me close

I close my eyes

And lean in for his kiss...

4 Sweetology & FrAnkenology
Understanding What's In YOUR Food
Sugar

Ok…we've arrived at the sticky part. I want to give you all of the good stuff, but sometimes, just sometimes, it's important to understand what hurts you so you can shift towards what heals you. As mentioned before, if you only get one thing from this book, learn to **read and question INGREDIENTS.** In this chapter about sugar and toxic and artificial foods, I will show you what happens when you start to question ingredients lurking in unsuspected places. As you read through the following pages, let this book act as your resource and a gentle friendly nudge, over and over again, to become an **Ingredientologist!**

Brace yourself. You know it's coming…that lecture that's gonna make you feel bad for all those sweet things that you love, enjoy, look forward to… yet deep down know they hurt you with that false illusion of momentary pleasure.

> *"The truth will set you free, but first it will piss you off."*
> *- Gloria Steinem*

So it's Halloween and I felt pretty smug about passing up every little packaged 'treat' and then got in my car, drove 20 minutes out of the way to find my 'Upgraded' - yet still refined - sugar fix. It had been a long time! Like any good addict, I was convinced I could do this just one more time, enjoy the benefits, and escape the consequences.

On my way to the post office, I often passed by a pastry shop with a faint auditory whimper. My intent as I walked inside, smothered by the smell of coffee and fresh baked pastries, was to get just ONE cinnamon roll. Instead, I walked out with two, sat in my car, snarfed down the first one… and literally as I reached into the bag for the second one I thought, where did the first one go? It didn't even taste as good as I built it up to be, but I was already gobbling down the second one. It had been a long time since I had refined sugar … sugar and gluten together… whowzah!

My class was 20 minutes away (thankfully, I was not teaching it) and after five minutes, I knew my day was over and I had to go home. I had forgotten about the severe brain fog (funny about that forgetfulness), and then my agitation set in and I knew I was done for the day. Like a zombie, I plunked myself in front of the computer and watched movie after movie. I white knuckled my way through the night so that I didn't go out again and find more 'fixes'.

Sounds like someone on drugs or an alcoholic, eh? Sugar is a drug, a legal, sell it solo, or by the dozen and pound drug. Don't believe me? Sugar has been said to be as addictive as cocaine! Refined sugar's sweetness is deceptive and always has been. You may experience some or many of these side-effects without realizing their link to sugar consumption.

Side Effects of Refined Sugar

* Disrupts your body's homeostasis (state of harmony and balance).
* Depletes and interferes with the absorption of essential minerals (i.e. calcium and magnesium) and nutrients in the body. Renders many vitamins and supplements useless. Sugar will utilize nutrients for its own metabolism and reduces the effectiveness of expensive supplements.
* Decreases the body's ability to fight off bacterial infections and infectious diseases. Most people believe that the flu comes around every year, but sugar makes a good host for "those bugs" which depletes the immune system. Maybe it's not the 'flu' – it's probably the refined sugar!
* Allergies - the more sugar and processed frankenfoods you have in your body, the more you are susceptible to allergies.
* Loss of tissue elasticity in our skin – increases wrinkles and premature aging.
* Biggest cause of ADD & ADHD – we would see miraculous improvement in school performance if kids did not consume refined sugar, which includes sodas and colorful drinks.
* Linked to the cause and feeding of cancer – lowers the immune system's natural ability to stay strong.
* Linked with alcoholism – alcohol and sugar create similar symptoms in the body, and both are extremely addictive substances.
* Eyes are more susceptible to macular degeneration and other eye and visual problems.
* Can cause hypoglycemia, pre-diabetes, type II diabetes, and gestational diabetes.
* Major contributing factor of fatigue, depression and fibromyalgia.
* Contributes to Alzheimer's and dementia – link between high blood sugar and Alzheimer's. Some doctors are calling Alzheimer's -Type 3 Diabetes!
* Produces acidity in the system.
* Causes tooth decay and periodontal disease.
* Contributes to obesity and the inability to lose weight.
* Not a complete list.

Before you feel your life is over and think I'm going to suggest that you remove all sugar from your life, just know that whatever I suggest to delete/alter I offer a better, healthier Upgrade for you! Upgraded Sweeteners don't have the same negative effects as refined sugar. You **can** indulge in Upgraded Sweeteners without the above symptoms. So stay with me here… this is the important stuff.

Sugar is hidden in sport drinks, energy drinks, fruit juices, and fast foods/processed foods --everything from lunch meat to sauces to cheese! Horrifically, it's even found in most infant formulas. Did you know that many infant formulas have as much sugar as a soda?!?!

* **The average 12 ounce soda has about 39 grams of refined sugar!!!**

Many people drink a LOT of soda. A 32 ounce soda has about 91 grams of refine sugar. Even worse, this sugar is mostly in the form of high fructose corn syrup, which is highly processed. High fructose corn syrup comes from GMO corn. According to Dr. Hyman, MD, high fructose corn syrup (HFCS) contains mercury that is not regulated or measured by the FDA.

Sugar & The Dangers of Food Marketing

Why is sugar so prominent at schools, malls, community functions, hospitals, offices and in peoples' refrigerators? As mentioned before, it all comes down to marketing and advertising. They do a great job of convincing us not to look under the hood at the ingredients, and to just focus on the smiling, beautiful people they have on their billboards, TV commercials, and packaging. Don't believe me? Look at the ingredients of foods that celebrities promote. Do the research for yourself – you will be shocked!

I think the sugar companies own holidays… what do you think? Every holiday is another opportunity to sell SUGAR. Holidays are riddled with oh, just have fun, give in, indulge… it's about food which means it's about love and laughter and happiness (so the commercials and packages show us). This was not the intent of the real holidays. Is Christmas really supposed to be about stuffing yourself with refined sugar and GMO frankenfoods, and then sitting on the couch drooling from brain fog? The origins behind Thanksgiving and the fall harvest does not mean picking up processed, chemical-filled foods at the grocery store. Halloween did not begin with popular brands of mini GMO-filled junk food to keep kids awake with a stomachache all night. Then there's Easter. How did we go from a pasture-raised egg that has nutrients to a chemically-laden chocolate egg that is full of refined sugar and processed gunk? Chocolate shaped Easter bunny? Sugary milk chocolate money for Chanukah! Oy Vey! Not to mention, SO much of this advertising is targeted towards impressionable kids.

Upgrade your thoughts: Begin to look at food commercials and advertising with a critical mind. Look at what they try to sell you and ask yourself: Do they care about my health or their profit? The words "nutritious" and "natural" are key words that large companies proudly advertise. They BANK on you TRUSTING them, and they BANK on you not questioning their ingredients. My jaw is on the floor every time I watch a commercial. Begin to really listen to the side effects of the medications advertised as well. I also encourage you to go to the store and read the ingredients on any of the foods advertised on TV. You just might be horrified.

We need a **TRUE** and **HONEST food education**. We have to make peace with ourselves, and peace with the foods we consume. This requires some research and the willingness to Upgrade. Fortunately, there are amazing people creating new and nourishing Upgrades that are available for just about everything you crave.

Processed & Packaged Foods - a.k.a. Frankenfoods

Sugar has many names and is found in most processed and packaged foods. Processed starches such as white flour, white rice, pasta (unless gluten-free whole grains), enriched flour, tapioca, cornstarch, and processed breakfast cereals have the same effect in your body as refined sugar. Refined sugar is added as a preservative because it increases the shelf life which increases profits. Always do your research and begin to read the INGREDIENTS and ask: **What's really in my food?** (Refer to Ch. 3, page 54).

So... remember to always read and ask about the Ingredients!

Use the list below and look at the foods in your pantry. Are you surprised to find refined sugar in some of them?

One way to find Refined Sugar is to look for anything that ends in OSE:

* Sucr**ose**
* Malt**ose**
* Dextr**ose**

* Fruct**ose (HFCS)**
* Gluc**ose**
* Galact**ose**

* Lact**ose**
* Gluc**ose** Solids
* Sucr**ose**

SOME of the other names that sugar is hidden under:

* Agave
* Barley Malt
* Beet Sugar
* Brown Sugar
* Buttered Syrup
* Cane Juice
* Caramel
* Castor Sugar
* Concentrated Fruit
* Corn Sweetener
* Corn Syrup
* Corn Syrup Solids
* Carob Syrup
* Crystalline
* D-Mannose
* Demerara
* Dextrin
* Dextran
* Dextrose
* Diastatic Malt

* Diastase
* Ethyl Maltol
* Evaporated Cane Juice
* Free Flowing
* Florida Crystals
* Fructose
* Fruit Juice
* Fruit Juice
  Concentrate
* Galactose
* Glucose
* Glucose Solids
* Golden Sugar
* Golden Syrup
* Grape Juice
* High Fructose Corn
  Syrup
* HFCS
* Honey (Unless Raw)
* Jaggery

* Lactose
* Maltodextrin
* Maltose
* Malt Syrup
* Mannitol
* Muscovado
  Sugar
* Panocha
* Rapundra
* Raw Sugar
* Refiner's Syrup
* Rice Syrup
* Sorbitol
* Sorghum Syrup
* Sucanat
* Sucrose
* Treacle

NOT a complete list

After going through your kitchen, were you surprised by how much refined sugar (and other chemicals) you consume on a daily basis? Imagine removing sugar from your life -- sounds painful, right? But wait! Don't go cold turkey! There are Upgraded Sugars available to you that are delicious and satisfying! Upgrade slowly, or you will experience detox symptoms that will probably lead you right back to these foods you are trying to Upgrade from (see How to Detox from Sugar, on page 76).

Do you have any symptoms that could be possibly related to refined sugars?

Check off any symptoms that you currently experience:

- ☐ Hormone Issues
- ☐ Constant infections (yeast or Candida)
- ☐ Skin issues, eczema
- ☐ Do you catch every cold and flu?
- ☐ Allergies
- ☐ ADD or ADHD, trouble concentrating?
- ☐ Brain Fog
- ☐ Cancer
- ☐ Alcoholism
- ☐ Hypoglycemic

- ☐ Diabetic
- ☐ Serious vision problems
- ☐ Fatigue, chronic fatigue
- ☐ Depression
- ☐ Fibromyalgia
- ☐ Early onset dementia or Alzheimer's
- ☐ Acidic stomach
- ☐ Excessive tooth decay or periodontal disease
- ☐ Obese or the inability to lose excess weight

Dr. Weston A. Price, a dentist in the 1920's, traveled the world to find out what factors contributed to tooth decay. He found that people who had major teeth problems and teeth/jaw deformities also suffered from major illnesses. He conducted his research by living in remote villages in Alaska, Switzerland and Africa. He found that once refined sugar was added into the villagers' diets, their health began to decline. He found that remote villages (that were not attached by roads to the bigger villages) were not exposed to sugar. As a result, he found that these remote villagers had nearly perfect health and beautiful, straight white teeth (and they did not have dentists, fluoride, braces, or tooth brushes… that's something to chew on). Dr. Price's research shows that it makes a lot of sense to gradually Upgrade from refined sugars in your life!

What would your life look like if you had delicious and nourishing sweetened treats without having to experience the side effects from refined sugars?

Are you willing to Upgrade?

When your body doesn't receive real food and nutrients, then your body goes into starvation mode. In this mode, it stores everything for 'emergencies'. This storage is the poundage we put on year after year and diet after diet.

You will feel better once you begin to Upgrade and eat real foods, use Upgraded sweeteners, and release the toxic and fake foods. As a result, your body will regulate, cravings will gradually subside, and your body will naturally release ailments and weight.

You are emotionally connected to the foods you enjoy eating (see Cravings on page 35). The good news is that you don't have to give up these foods when you learn to Upgrade them. Upgrading is that win-win solution. These pages are full of creative and delicious possibilities just waiting for you.

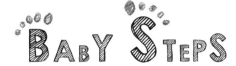

 **Identify foods and beverages in your home that CONTAIN refined sugars:**

 **Take your favorite sugary item and review the UPGRADES.**
Find Upgrades in Chapter 6 (page 132) or Recipe Alterations on page 150 to alter it:

 **Once you Upgrade your favorite sugary item, make sure to keep plenty of the Upgraded item on hand so you feel SATISFIED by it:**

Note: If you are not satisfied at first with your Upgrade, alter the recipe or try another option. **Get creative** and **curious** until you find something that **tastes delicious and satisfies you**. If you are still tempted by the old version over your new one, see what you can do to enhance it just a little bit more. **You want to get to a point where your Upgraded version tastes so good and satisfies you completely.** When this happens, it's less likely that you will fall back to that old version. This is SO important to understand. **If you don't find something that completely satisfies you - it's more likely that the old version will find its way back into your belly when you least expect it.**

The Scary on Artificial Sweeteners - a.k.a. Frankenfoods

"Our natural ability to control how much we eat and, therefore, our body weight may be weakened when this natural link is impaired by consuming products that contain artificial sweeteners." - Natasha Turner, ND

Artificial sweeteners are TOXIC CHEMICALS and they are cheap to produce. The marketing pros know how to lure in the dieters, the calorie counters, and people who have diabetes and weight issues. If you see something that says 'zero-calories', 'reduced calories', 'fat-free', 'non-fat' and basically claim diet food status, you will very likely find artificial sweeteners and chemicals in them.

You may *think* artificial sweeteners are better than refined sugar, but they are not – they are far, far worse. Artificial sweeteners come with serious side effects, and create toxicity and confusion in your body. When combining artificial sweeteners and artificial colors, these fake foods become more toxic and negatively affect your brain and neurological function. Food "facts" may claim zero to very few calories in artificial sweeteners, but this comes at the expense of tricking your body.

According to Dr. Mark Hyman, people who go on diets (usually diets that encourage eating low-fat, fat-free and artificially sweetened foods) GAIN back on average 11 pounds for every diet they follow! These toxic chemicals SLOW DOWN your metabolism and STORE FAT, while losing muscle.

Artificial sweeteners desensitize your taste buds. When your taste buds taste sweet foods, the body releases a hormone called insulin (just as if you actually had sugar). Insulin makes the blood sugar rise and increases your cravings. This leaves you feeling hungrier which leads to eating more and more! Many people who ingest artificial sweeteners tend to GAIN MORE weight compared to regular sugar because it confuses the body's signals. Artificial foods are not nearly as satisfying as the nourishing food that contains real ingredients.

There are thousands and thousands of so-called food items with artificial sweeteners in them. Here are a just a handful of possibilities where you will find artificial sweeteners. Artificial sweeteners are found in over 6,000 items! **YIKES!**

These are just a few items LOADED with Artificial Sweeteners:

* Bottled drinks & sodas
* Powdered drinks
* Gum
* Pastries
* Gelatins
* Dessert mixes
* Puddings
* Fillings
* Frozen desserts
* Yogurt
* Chewable vitamins
* Sugar-free products
* Diet foods/zero or low calorie drinks
* And so on...

Artificial Sweeteners can also be found under these names:

* Acesulfame-K
* Aspartame
* Equal®
* NutraSweet®
* Saccharin
* Sweet'n Low®
* Sucralose
* Splenda®
* Sorbitol
* Neotame

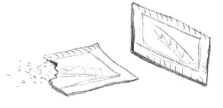

Not-So-Sweet Effects of Artificial Sweeteners

Some artificial sweeteners have been linked to cancer, headaches, dizziness, hallucinations and metabolic issues. 10% of aspartame will breakdown into methanol (wood alcohol). The EPA says a safe consumption of methanol is about 7.8 milligrams per day which equals about 6 oz. of diet soda. I know people who drink 64 ounces of this poison daily! This concoction that passes through the system with pectin (a fiber) will create formaldehyde in the system. Formaldehyde (paint remover, embalming fluid, etc.) creates cancer in the human system. Formaldehyde in the system can also create acidosis (excessive acidity in the blood). As a result, this can create blindness, kidney damage, organ failure, etc. **Ugh!**

Some documented symptoms associated with aspartame:

* Headaches
* Moodiness
* Vision changes
* Convulsions/seizures
* Sleep Issues
* Insomnia
* Change in heart rate
* Hallucinations

* Abdominal cramps or pain
* Memory loss
* Rash
* Nausea or vomiting
* Fatigue or weakness
* Poor equilibrium/dizziness
* Diarrhea
* Hives

* Joint pain
* Depression
* Cancer
* Not a complete list

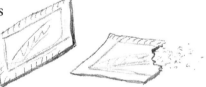

Artificial Sweeteners create WEIGHT Gain (as mentioned above). Aspartame releases hormones in the body that **DIRECT** the body to **STORE FAT**. It also **turns off your 'full' signal**, much like MSG (monosodium glutamate - think Chinese food). And this creates MORE food cravings. Think about what it's like to drive with your emergency brake on. How long until that unpleasant burning smell starts to happen? That burning smell is your symptom. Take the brake off (take out the artificial sweeteners) and the smell (side effects) begins to go away.

Research shows that the first artificial sweetener was discovered in 1878 by a chemist working with a carcinogenic material - coal tar. Yup, the first sweetener was produced out of coal tar. Say What?!!

Drinking **diet soda INCREASES** your **risk of diabetes** and is murder on the system of a diabetic. It still boggles my mind that most diabetic food plans include a slew of artificial, low-fat, fat-free ingredients. **The fat is not the problem**; the problem is the kind of fat and where it originates.

A study conducted at the University of Texas showed that people who drink diet sodas are 65% more likely to be overweight than people who do not drink any soda. They are also more likely to be overweight than people who drink regular soda. Even though the high fructose corn syrup in soda is horrible, diet sodas and fake sugars are far, far worse.

Ask yourself this question: Do you know someone who drinks a lot of diet drinks and eats a lot of diet, non-fat or low-fat foods and is still very overweight? IF these 'Diet' foods really worked, wouldn't people who consume them be at their ideal weight?

How to Upgrade from Artificial Sweeteners

Start with just one item that you eat or drink that contains artificial sweeteners. If you still feel you must have your low/no-calorie sweetener, then switch to organic green powder stevia. Hint: the white stevia is still refined even though it's the only one available in packets at this time. The green powder stevia is usually found in the bulk sections at natural food stores. When switching over to an organic brand of the white stevia, it's still considered an Upgrade from artificial sweeteners.

 Identify any foods or drinks that you currently enjoy that have artificial ingredients in them. Ask yourself, **WHY** do you use them? Is it for weight loss? If so, know that **artificial sweeteners create weight GAIN**! Is it for the taste and texture? If so, it has probably been a long time since you ate/drank the real deal and it's tainted your taste buds.

 Use the Upgrades or Recipe Alteration Charts on page 150 to Upgrade this item.

 Keep altering the item until it tastes satisfying and delicious to you (so that you won't be tempted to go back to the frankenfoods)!

Begin to think about Upgrades in the 'stranded desert island' analogy. **Make the most nourishing decision possible with what you have**. If I were stranded on a desert island and there were only 3 native coconuts left, 1 candy bar, a case of diet soda, 1 box of Grandma's homemade cookies and 2 bottles of fruit juice – this is how I would navigate it.

1st - Native land food: I'd make the coconuts last as long as possible – hoping to be rescued before I had to move onto the next items.
2nd - Grandma's cookies (OK! I'd probably indulge in these since I'm stranded on a desert island)
3rd - Fruit Juice
4th - Candy Bar
5th - I'd personally try to filter the ocean water through rocks and drink that before the diet soda (because of my negative history with artificial sweeteners).

This may be a far-fetched example, but **think about real life and the choices you make every day.** The closest thing to this would be the convenience store while on a road trip. For example, you go over a big bump and your cooler full of all your amazing Upgrades falls off the truck without you knowing… what would you do? If your only option is a convenience store, walk around and figure out what is the best possible food (with the cleanest ingredients) that you can eat - with what you have available in that moment.

So how do you feel about Artificial Sweeteners now? You may feel a little lost at this moment because if you made the switch from regular sugar to artificial sweeteners, it's probably due to the many downfalls of refined sugar. Let's look at the next section of Upgraded Sweeteners for your best Upgraded options, which I promise are tasty and nutritious!

How to Detox from Sugar Without Biting Off Someone's Head

Unless you add in the nourishing, Upgraded Sweeteners that are listed on the next page, you WILL experience symptoms and signs of DETOX from releasing sugar.

Detox signs may include some of the following:
* Fatigue
* Headache
* Moodiness
* Moderate to Intense cravings
* Feeling like you are white knuckling / using all your willpower
* Failure to keep from eating that sworn off food
* Dehydration
* Aches and Pains
* Brain Fog

Refined sugar was designed to keep you hooked so that you give into your craving. Think of sugar as a drug addiction - it takes time to detox from drugs. Therefore, it takes time to detox from the sugar. It takes about two weeks to get refined sugar out of your system. The first few days can be difficult **IF** you don't replace it with Upgraded Sweeteners.

It's the diet mentality that tells us to get rid of the foods we love, which includes sugar. This all-or-nothing mentality usually leads us right back to sugar or to artificial sugars. If you find yourself face first in the sweets during the next holiday (or the next time someone waves sugar in front of your nose), then return to this section and try another sugar alternative. Trust me on this one!

"The key to success is failure." - Michael Jordan

Remember

If you only get three things out of this book:

1. Read ALL Ingredients!

2. Take an inventory of the foods you love!

3. Upgrade the ingredients!

Upgrades for
Refined Sugar & Artificial Sweeteners

Upgrade from chemically processed, artificial sweeteners in packets or in processed foods. Read the ingredients because many of them use wording such as 'All Natural'. Begin to try some of these Upgraded Sweeteners until you feel **satisfied**.

Low Glycemic

(Beneficial if you have issues regulating your blood sugar levels)

* Organic Berries
* Organic Coconut Sugar / Coconut Palm Sugar
* Organic Green Stevia Powder
* Organic Sweet Vegetables such as Carrots, Sweet Potatoes, etc.
* Low Glycemic fruits such as Grapefruit, Lemon, Lime and Berries

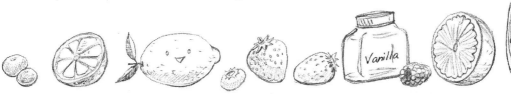

Upgrades for Refined Sugar & Artificial Sweeteners

* Organic Coconut Sugar /Coconut Palm Sugar
* Organic Coconut Nectar
* Organic RAW Honey (local if possible)
* Organic Grade B Maple Syrup
* Organic Date Syrup
* Organic Dried Fruits
* Organic Fruit

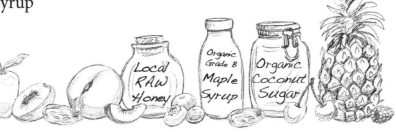

NOTE: Most **Agave nectar** is now processed like **high fructose corn syrup**, and is high in fructose and **difficult for the liver to process**. True Agave Nectar is CLEAR. If you must have it, then Upgrade to the best Agave Nectar possible. Read labels and research before you purchase items with sweeteners you are not familiar with. If you do not have any blood sugar issues, you may be able to tolerate Agave as an Upgrade from refined sugar. However, if you have any blood sugar issues, I recommend Upgrades from lists above.

More **Upgraded Sweeteners** can be found on pages 77, 83-85.

How to Upgrade from Refined and Artificial Sugar

Drink lots of purified water

Water assists in cleaning out the toxins. As mentioned before, it takes about two weeks to get rid of refined sugar and other toxins from your body. But it's worth it so give it a two week trial.

A lack of water leads to dehydration which can lead to cravings for sweets. Drink a glass of water 20 minutes before eating (especially if one of those little sugary guys call out to you). Stop, drink water, and take a few deep breaths. See Cravings in Chapter 2 (page 46) on how to increase water intake.

Start your day with breakfast (see Breakfast ideas on page 112). Always eat a nutritious and Upgraded breakfast to get you started and set the tone of your day.

Eat lots of fresh and sweet vegetables

Sweet veggies such as carrots, parsnips, jicama, and sweet potatoes give you a sense of sweetness and fullness. The more often you consume sweet vegetables, the less you'll crave refined sugar.

Eat fresh fruit

Fruits are healthy, delicious, full of fiber, nutrients, and sweetness. Eat fresh fruit and avoid fruit juices or concentrates. All store bought fruit juices have been processed through pasteurization (heat) and no longer have the natural enzymes to break down the sugar. This turns fruit juices into pure sugar. Fruit juice also spikes insulin and creates a roller coaster imbalance for your blood sugar and liver.

Add some organic nut butter (read ingredients on all nut butters – I currently purchased one I thought was just sunflower seed butter and to my dismay it had sugar in it), nuts, or seeds to your fruit. This helps slow down the sugar going through your bloodstream. My clients have found that eating fruit alone creates more and more sugar cravings, but when they add some nut butter, nuts, or seeds that helps slow down cravings and makes their snack more satisfying. Refer to Slow Carbs/Fast Carbs and Magic Trio Combinations (page 101) for more information.

Upgrade from fat-free or low-fat processed snack foods

Real food is real good, while fake foods fake out your body! Fat-free, low-fat and processed franken-foods mostly contain high quantities of refined sugar or artificial sweeteners to compensate for lack of flavor and fat. This sends your blood sugar on a roller coaster of highs and lows. They also contain artificial flavorings which can lead to neurological issues and to more of the artificial or refined sweet stuff. These foods trick your body and make you gain weight and crave more foods…the exact opposite of why you buy them.

Experiment with spices

Coriander, cinnamon, nutmeg, cloves, and cardamom will naturally sweeten your foods to help reduce cravings. See **Upgrades** (starting on page 131) for more ideas.

Snacks

Snack often! Keep Upgraded snacks with you to avoid your blood sugar dropping. If you have a snack BEFORE your blood sugar drops, you can keep it regulated and you won't worry about what you need to eat to raise your blood sugar! I suggest snacking at least every 2-3 hours so you don't get too hungry.

> **Once you reach that very hungry place it's difficult to make healthy decisions.** As a result, your body goes into panic mode because your blood sugar has dropped. Once your blood sugar has dropped too low, you will reach for the first thing that promises to increase your energy again. This is usually sugar and/or caffeine. Don't let the blood sugar monster get ya! Check out back-up snacks and the **"Gotta Go Bag"** in Chapter 5 on page 118.

Stress Relief

Let's go back to what I mentioned about cravings. Your cravings are often created by your emotions. Add in the *low blood sugar monster* and this wreaks havoc in your body.

If under pressure, try one of the following:

* Drink a glass of water
* Take a walk
* Take a deep breath
* Step outside
* Look around your environment
* Count backwards from 10 to 1, taking a deep breath with each count
* Get in the car and scream or Shake, Shake, Shake your body!
  See Movement Section in Chapter 9, pages 208 & 212.

Sugar Questions:

? What is your relationship with refined sugar?

? What if removing refined sugar from your life would relieve most or all of your symptoms? Would you make a sincere effort to try it for two weeks?

? If so, what do you need to do to make this transition successful?

? What is your resistance (if any) to Upgrading your sweeteners for two weeks?

? What kind of obstacles could get in your way of this success (foods people bring home, into the office, restaurant/café temptations, free food etc.)?

? If the obstacles are vast... what is **one** item that you eat daily that you could **Upgrade**?

Slow down, you say? Sure!

Start with just one item you eat and crave and begin to Upgrade just that product. Make sure to find a clean and nourishing ingredient alternative that satisfies you. Play around with the recipe or try different products until you find the one that's just right (Goldilocks at the grocery store, reading labels, tasting, too sweet, not sweet enough, too chalky …ahhhhh just right).

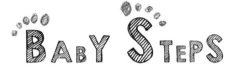

Pick just ONE of the steps from the previous page to begin.
Recommendation: Water (See Water section on page 46):

Pick one more of the steps and begin to incorporate.
Recommendation: Snacks (See Snacks on page 114 for more options):

Pick a third step from above and incorporate.
Recommendation: Start with a healing breakfast.
(See Breakfast section on page 112 for more options):

The Banana Versus the Pancake

Many years ago I went to my parents' home for a visit. We had just gone out to breakfast where my father, a diabetic of 13 years, had pancakes and syrup. Nothing healthy, just your typical chain restaurant. The worst possible ingredients in those pancakes and syrup included white flour, refined sugar, high fructose corn syrup (it's never real Maple Syrup in a restaurant unless listed), fake egg products, coloring, flavoring…yaddah, yaddah, yaddah.

After breakfast, we arrived back at their house. I was sorting through my luggage and offered my father the organic bananas I had with me. My father - without flinching - said, "No, I can't have bananas because of my diabetes!" I looked at him and "But those pancakes and syrup are diabetic friendly, eh!" just slipped out of my mouth. He did a double take (touché), shook his head at the situation, and tried to explain how the pancakes and syrup were a once in a while treat.

So to get this story straight. He 'saved up' his 'treat' of pancakes and syrup which are devoid of nutrients, full of refined sugar, and pure aggravation in the system of a diabetic - instead of eating something natural, delicious, and full of fiber and nutrients (he likes bananas). He would be better off with five banana's every day or Upgraded Pancakes (see page 231) rather than those refined sugar, chemical filled pancakes and syrup once a week.

Your thoughts?

Where do you fall into this story?

Giving up something natural, such as fruit (because it has natural sugar) OR opting for an over the top sugary treat that harms you? Please take this story to heart. When you want something sweet, see if something natural, such as fruit or Upgraded Sweeteners will satisfy you first.

The next step? You got it…Upgrade to the cleanest quality ingredients you can!

How can you tell if refined sugars linger in your food? Refer back to **Ingredientology** on page 53, and begin to **research the ingredients you don't understand.**

What are FrAnKenFoods

Let's dive into what lurks in those processed, brightly packaged foods, and fast foods and drinks that we eat way too often. As I said before, there are many chemicals and fake ingredients in foods these days that it can be overwhelming sometimes. I'm going to share a few of them so you can start thinking about what it is inside your food. It's important to start reading ingredients (refer to Ingredientology on page 53). For now, let's go over some of the muggers out there.

"People are gaining weight today because they eat too much chemically-processed, artificial junk food and consume too much caffeine, sugar, nicotine, and alcohol. It's not the carbohydrates."
-Joshua Rosenthal, Institute for Integrative Nutrition

Food companies come up with new products and different names for refined sugar and chemicals all the time. Years ago, the name list was at 80 and in late 2014, it's at 312 and increasing! The foods you probably consume are packaged and processed foods. These are extremely convenient, usually quite inexpensive, AND have a long shelf or refrigerator life due to preservatives. The additives help make the foods taste better and look better. However, they are far more expensive than the price tag. The side-effects alone add up to various ailments and diseases. As I reminded you in previous sections, your first step is to KNOW what's inside the foods you eat.

Become familiar with the side effects and see if any of them apply to you. Start with the food that you eat most and Upgrade that one. If you need to go slower, start with a once in a while food that feels good to Upgrade. Start with something. Every little baby step you take improves your health and well-being.

Give yourself an Alternative so that you can remove the Refined SUGAR and other harmful chemicals found in so many foods, but keep that sweet flavor that you LOVE.

Create a list of options and keep it with you at all times so you can know and weigh out the healthier alternatives!
(See I Can list Ch 8, page 182 / My Upgrades list in Ch 6, page 150).

Be gentle and kind with yourself! Look for the sweetness and the savory in life. Ask yourself: is it mouth hunger or emotional hunger? How would you treat a child? Don't beat yourself up! Notice how the food affects you, and find an Upgrade for your 'next time'.
Keep coming back to what you CAN DO!

Upgraded Sweeteners

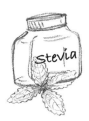

Organic Green Powder Stevia (it's GREEN, not the white stuff) is a South American herb/plant. Remember that your taste buds change once you get the refined sugars out of your system and you may discover at first you don't like the taste of stevia. After some time you may grow to enjoy it. Mix it with some coconut sugar, maple syrup or raw local honey to help make the transition easier.

Benefits: a healthful low glycemic sweetener and be found in either powder or liquid concentrate. One teaspoon of stevia is SWEETER than 1 cup of sugar. The real stuff is extremely sweet and will have an aftertaste.

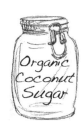

Organic Coconut Sugar or Coconut Palm Sugar is one of the lower glycemic sweeteners. It's made from the sap of the palm or coconut trees and is ground down and dehydrated. It has a lot of fiber and tastes delicious (similar to brown sugar). This type of sugar melts quickly and is easy to use. It can be substituted in recipes that call for sugar. Instead of **s'mores**, try this sweet treat instead. **Skewer peaches, apples or pears and then dip in cinnamon and coconut sugar!** Yum!

Benefits: It is a low glycemic sweetener and high in nutrients.

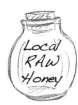

Organic Local Raw Honey is one of the oldest sweeteners that is made from bees pollinating flowers. It's fantastic to use in raw and baked desserts. Local raw honey has great benefits and can actually help with seasonal allergies and coughs! Add it to your sipping tea for sweetness.

Benefits: Full of nutrients and beneficial enzymes. Excellent for Allergies.

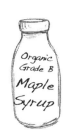

Organic Grade B Maple Syrup is from the sap of the maple trees. I recommend using Grade B maple syrup. It's slightly darker and has higher minerals. The lighter colored maple syrups, Grade A, are lighter because the trees have been tapped during a colder temperature and need less sap to boil into syrup. Grade B, or darker syrup, comes from maple trees tapped during warmer temperatures and more sap is needed to boil it into syrup. This increases the mineral contents of the sap. Organic is best because the trees have not been sprayed with any chemicals, which could contaminate the sap. Add it into anything that needs a little lightness to it such as cakes!

Benefits: Full of natural minerals and can even boost your immune system.

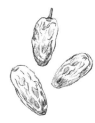

Organic Dates are natural, and full of nutrients and fiber. To use them, first soak them in water. You can soak them overnight in water in a jar – or soak them for a couple of hours then grind them up into a paste. You can also soak them for a full day and just use the liquid. Use instead of honey or agave. My favorite are Medjool dates!

Benefits: Full of nutrients and fiber!

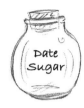

Organic Date Sugar is made from the pressing and dehydrating of dates. This is best used as a topping or an ingredient mixed with cinnamon or crumb topping since it doesn't dissolve very easily.

Benefits: Full of minerals (not as complete as using real dates but does have some of the nutrients).

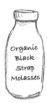

Organic Black Strap Molasses Full of minerals. Combine with lower glycemic sweeteners and use for things like ginger bread, cookies or cakes.

Benefits: It contains enzymes, iron, magnesium, selenium, potassium and copper.

Lacuma is a fruit from South America. It has a slightly maple flavor and tastes great in smoothies or baked goods.

Benefits: High in antioxidants, low glycemic, and full of beta-carotenes and Vitamin B.

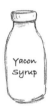

Yacon is an extract from the Yacon plant, a tuberous root. It's found in Bolivia, Brazil and Peru. It's considered a 'designer sweetener' because it's more expensive. It has a slightly maple and earthy flavor to it.

Benefits: High in fiber and low glycemic.

Here are some great Upgrades that you can use to sweeten your foods:

Unsweetened applesauce is a great way to replace white sugar and is a good Upgrade in a pinch! It can be replaced one for one in most baking recipes, or take it a step further by making your own applesauce. When you buy applesauce in the store, it's been heat pasteurized. Pasteurization kills naturally occurring enzymes which assists with the preservation of food. This is why canned and jarred foods have long shelf lives.

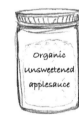

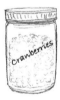

Cranberries are another type of sweet and tart food that can be added to food for a bit of zing. Be sure to get unsweetened and use your own Upgraded Sweeteners. Bonus: cranberries help alleviate urinary tract infections. Use for things like ginger bread, cookies or cakes.

Bananas can also be used as substitutes for some sweets. A frozen banana can be blended into the consistency of soft serve ice cream for a sweet treat. As bananas ripen, the natural sugars in the fruit increase.

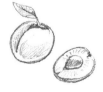

Apricot Puree is easy to make and makes a sweet syrup. It's full of Vitamin C, fiber, and iron. To make the puree, soak dried apricots in water, blend, and strain. This can be done with most dried fruits, but make sure to use organic fruits without any additives. If your fruit has added sulfur or concentrates, it's just as processed as a food filled with sugar.

Freshly Squeezed Juices are great and healthy alternatives to bottled fruit drinks. Use fresh squeezed fruits. If you find that making your own juice is too messy or time consuming, consider trying out a juice bar. Many of the larger health food stores have a juice bar (most 'Freshly Squeezed Juices' in the store are pasteurized, therefor lacking enzymes and are pure fructose/sugar).

Orange Zest adds a wonderful zing! Check out the recipe section for **Almond Biscotti** (page 262). Be prepared for yum—they're tasty and have a great crunch texture!

Spices can enhance the flavors in your food too!

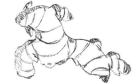

* Ginger
* Nutmeg
* Ceylon Cinnamon

* Cloves
* Cardamom
* Vanilla

What do you think of these Upgraded Sweeteners?

Hopefully, you no longer feel deprived because, as you can see, there are many ingredients to choose from to help satisfy your sweet tooth. **Don't forget about fruits and sweet vegetables. Make sure to check out the Fiber, Protein, and Fat section (Chapter 5, page 104)** to make sure you metabolize them efficiently without leading to cravings.

How to Make Your Own Liquid Stevia

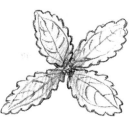

Ingredients
* ¼ cup organic green stevia powder (or dry and grind up stevia leaves)
* 1 cup hot purified water

Directions:
1. In a glass jar, stir together the stevia and hot water.
2. Let it cool at room temperature (2-4 hours).
3. If you use the powder, strain and transfer the stevia into a dropper bottle for convenient use and then store it in the refrigerator.
4. If you use ground up leaves, strain the liquid before placing in the dropper bottle and refrigerator.
5. If you want more flavor, add a vanilla bean or extract of your choice (read ingredients on extracts).

Because alcohol is the most refined sugar, if you use extracts and are very sugar/alcohol sensitive you can gently boil the extract to remove the alcohol.

There are pure organic vanilla powders on the market that you can buy (READ the ingredients because many add sugar and other undesirables). You can add 1/8-1/4 tsp vanilla powder to your hot stevia liquid and let both cool to room temperature.

Questionable Sweeteners

Sweetened Fruit Juice is not recommended because they don't contain juice from organic fruits (unless it says organic). Grapes are usually the top ingredient for items that are fruit juice sweetened. Non-organic grapes are highly exposed to pesticides.

Barley Malt - Barley is Glutenous! It's not very sweet, but you'll find it in foods that say they are "grain-sweetened".

Agave - Controversy! Is not the best choice because it's mostly fructose and has to be metabolized by the liver. Fructose creates stress in your body. Most agave is highly processed. If you want to use agave, buy a pure, agave that is CLEAR! Agave does NOT have more nutrients the 'darker' it is. It is nothing like maple syrup.

Sucanat and Florida Cane Crystals are less refined than sugar cane, and have a trace amount of minerals and nutrients in the crystals but there are better alternatives. In the beginning, you can use these in recipes to replaced refined sugar. Use the same amount as you would for regular sugar. An even better option: use Coconut Sugar or Coconut Palm Sugar.

Brown Sugar is white refined sugar with some added molasses. Use Coconut Sugar instead.

Dextrose, Fructose and Glucose are simple sugars that are difficult for the liver to process. They are sweeter than sugar and have less calories (why they are included in 'diet' foods). They wreck havoc on your body. They can cause bloating, diarrhea and the farts!

Items made with sucralose (any of the packet artificial sweeteners) are in a similar boat as aspartame and saccharin, which cause numerous ill effects. Again, if you are still convinced that you need zero calorie and zero glycemic - go with organic GREEN stevia powder (most white stevia is highly processed).

Xylitol is not tolerated well by everyone because it works as a laxative. It's natural, but not meant for absorption so it passes through the small intestines un-digested. It's acceptable in gum, toothpaste, or mouthwash. If you want a non-caloric/zero glycemic sweetener choose organic green stevia powder.

I was working at a raw vegan retreat center when someone gave me a large homemade sesame seed bar. She told me it was just pressed sesame seeds, xylitol and sea salt. I thought how wonderful and proceeded to gobble it down. It was very sweet and extremely delicious. Within about 30 minutes, I had uncontrollable gas. It's a good thing I had my own office at the time. My stomach was a wreck for a couple of days.

Because my food was so clean at the time, it was obvious that my stomach havoc was from the xylitol. The good thing is that I have not had the desire for xylitol ever again! Not everyone had the same experience as I did with the xylitol. As mentioned before, some people can tolerate things that others cannot. Now I use stevia if I'm looking for a zero-glycemic sweetener.

Use Upgraded Sweeteners whenever possible, see pages 77, 83-85.

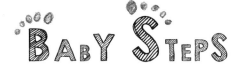

BABY STEPS

Decide to taste at least one of the Upgraded Sweeteners.
Which one?

Begin to use your favorite Upgraded Sweeteners in place of refined sugar or artificial sweeteners. Describe:

Allow yourself to indulge in your new favorite sweetener for at least 2 weeks. This will give you a chance to detox from refined sugars and/or artificial sweeteners. This will help you from feeling deprived. Feeling satisfied will assist you in releasing and upgrading from toxic and harmful sweeteners:

REMEMBER: Read ingredients and look out for hidden sugar and artificial sweeteners.

Learn more about **Sugar and Food Addictions** in Chapter 9, page 226.

ToXic and Fake Food-Like-Stuff

In my early 20s, I started getting wrist pains. Within a short amount of time, they got worse and worse. I saw a doctor who mentioned that it could be carpal tunnel syndrome so I researched more information about carpal tunnel. I knew a few people who also had carpal tunnel, but most were much older than me which concerned me even more. The notion of surgery to fix it was thrown around. I found that even people who had the surgery were not necessarily relieved of their pain, and they had more issues after the surgery.

An art teacher led me to an acupuncturist who didn't tell me much but gave me a list of foods to avoid. I was a bit shocked when I looked at the list because I realized that I consumed most of the items. These items were causing my inflammation. The biggest thing that I released was diet soda. I later learned that it was the artificial sweeteners in them that caused a lot of my pain and inflammation. A few years later I was pain free, and I decided that enough time had passed so I decided that a sip of soda wouldn't hurt. After one drink, the pain returned in minutes (a shooting pain down my wrist into my hands). After that painful experience, I made it a point to never have artificial sweeteners and I don't miss them one bit.

Artificial ingredients trick our bodies! Notice all the diet, low-fat, fat-free and gluten-free products in the market these days? As I mentioned earlier in the chapter, manufacturers are brilliant in their attempt to market frankenfoods to consumers. But you really don't know what's in that frankenfood, despite the misleading wording and packaging, until you read the ingredients. They figure that people won't read or understand the INGREDIENTS.

Upgrades from FrAnkenfoods

Dairy

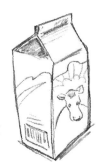

If you want/need/can't live without your dairy, be sure to get Organic and look for Grass Fed/Grass Finished. Otherwise, you will ingest hormones into your body that are meant for a one ton cow. Buy the real stuff and not the diet stuff (diet will be pumped full of artificial flavors/colors/sweeteners and artificial preservatives). Current studies show that Soy is no longer a beneficial alternative to dairy (see next page).

Dairy Upgrade Alternatives: Goat, Sheep, Coconut, Nuts and Seeds.

✳ Most Nourishing	Middle Ground	TOXIC
* Organic Grass Fed/Pasture Raised Raw Milk	* Organic Milk	✘ Regular Milk
* Organic Raw Sheep Milk	* Sheep/Goat Milk	✘ Non-Fat, Low-Fat
* Organic Raw Goat Milk	* Unsweetened Nut or Seed Milk purchased in cartons	✘ Fat-Free
* Organic Homemade Nut or Seed Milk		✘ Refined Sweetened
		✘ Artificially Flavored
		✘ Fortified Vitamins

Note: Items sold in cartons have all kinds of preservatives in them, be sure to get one with the minimal and most recognized ingredients or make your own.

Soy

Unless it says Organic & NON-GMO, then it's probably a frankenfood. Soy in abundance can cause damage to the thyroid and knock your hormones out of balance. I got onto the soy-boat as a young 20-year-old thinking I was being body-friendly. Because of soy, I believe it's one of the reasons why I still have a weight problem today. The thyroid is directly connected to the metabolism and our hormones, which dictates our weight.

Soy that is nourishing (in small amounts) is NON-GMO, Organic **fermented** soy products (see below). The cheap versions of soy/tamari sauce are made by a 24 hour, high heat chemical process. Real fermented food takes months (sometimes years) to ferment to perfection. You get what you pay for with QUALITY fermented foods.

Beware of Soy Oil! It's toxic and found in too many junk foods AND 'health food' products. Soy is extremely cheap to produce and is a very versatile crop.

Most Nourishing	Middle Ground	TOXIC
* Organic NON-GMO Fermented Soy Products * Tempeh, Miso, Natto, Tamari, Soy Sauce	* Organic NON-GMO * Soy Products	✗ Anything with Soy in it that is not Organic & NON-GMO ✗ Soy Oil is extremely toxic

Soy Alternative Upgrades

OLD	UPGRADED
Soy Sauce	Coconut Aminos
Soy Milk	Organic Nut, Seed or Coconut Milk
Soy Milk	Coconut Oil or Coconut Butter

Other names for soy found in foods:

* Bean Curd
* Edamame
* Hydrolyzed soy protein
* Kinnoko flour
* Kyodofu
* Lecithin (various spelling)
* Okara (soy pulp)
* Soy (anything with the name 'Soy' in it)
* Soya
* Soya Flour
* Soy Lecithin
* Soy Oil

* Soybean paste
* Supro
* Tamari
* Tempeh
* Teriyaki Sauce
* Textured soy flour (TSF)
* Textured soy protein (TSP)
* Textured vegetable protein (TVP)
* Tofu
* Yakidofu
* Yuba (bean curd)

Possible places where soy could be hidden:
* Vegetable, Plant or Bean in the name of something, unless it shows the source.
* Guar
* Xanathan
* Vitamin E
* Toccophernol
* MSG
* Natural & Artificial Flavor
* Mono-diglyceride
NOT a complete list

Corn

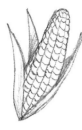

If you want corn, get Organic, NON-GMO Verified Corn. It is nutritious in it's original state. Otherwise it's probably GMO. If you are not familiar with GMO's and how they negatively affect our health and the environment, then I strongly encourage you to do your own research. Corn is an extremely versatile crop and below are JUST A FEW of the possible GMO Corn Products:

* Alcohol
* Artificial flavorings
* Artificial sweeteners
* Ascorbic acid (a.k.a FAKE Vitamin C)
* Aspartame
* Astaxanthin
* Baking powder
* Calcium citrate
* Carmel and carmel coloring
* Corn (anything)
* Dextrin/Dextrose
* Distilled white vinegar
* Glucosamine
* Glutamate
* Gluten feed/meal
* Golden syrup
* High Fructose Corn Syrup
* Hydrolyzed corn (anything)
* Hydrolyzed vegetable
* Invert syrup/sugar
* Lecithin
* Magnesium citrate/stearate
* Maize
* Malt syrup
* Manitol
* Maltodextrin
* Modified food starch
* MSG
* Natural flavorings
* Sucrose
* Treacle
* Vanilla/Vanillin
* Vitamin C / E
* **NOT a complete list**

Organic NON-GMO Popcorn

* 1/2 cup Organic Non-GMO Popcorn
* 1 TBSP Organic, Extra Virgin Coconut Oil

Option:
* 1 TBSP organic extra virgin coconut oil
* 3 drops stevia extract
* 1/2 tsp cinnamon
* Pinch of Celtic Sea Salt

Another Option:
* 1 TBSP organic extra virgin coconut oil
* 1/2 TBSP organic ground ginger
* 2 TBSP nutritional yeast

Directions:
1. Place 1/2-1 TBSP of organic extra virgin coconut oil in a pan with lid.
2. Place on medium heat and add just enough popcorn kernels to line the bottom of the pan.
3. Cover and wait for it to start popping. Once it's popping, let in a tiny bit of air if the lid does not have a steam release.
4. Once the popping starts to slow down, turn off stove and let the remainder pop.
5. After popcorn is popped, transfer to a bowl and sprinkle with 1-2 TBSP of nutritional yeast.

   Play with variations that you enjoy - get creative!

Wheat

The wheat we eat today is not like the wheat our ancestors ate. If you know you have issues with wheat, review the Upgrades chapter for more options. Unless the wheat says Organic and NON-GMO, it's Geneticlly Modified (also called GE for Genetically Engineered). Once again, I can't emphasize enough how important it is to read all ingredients!

Wheat Alternatives: There are some great gluten-free alternative grains available. However, they do not have the same texture, but they can still be satisfying. See chart below and Recipes in Appendix for more ideas.

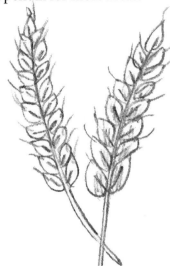

Warning: If you are sensitive to wheat, then you may also be sensitive to glutenous grains such as spelt, kamut, barley and rye.

If you have a **gluten sensitivity,** you may experience any of the following symptoms:

* Abdominal pain/discomfort such as bloating or gas
* Diarrhea or constipation/ Irritable bowel
* Headaches/Migraines
* Acne (more than just a few pimples)
* Fatigue/Lethargy
* Inflammation such as bone or joint pain

If you have any of these reactions after eating gluten, then you may have a gluten intolerance and I urge you to **Upgrade to Organic, NON-GMO Gluten-Free Grains**.

Gluten-Free

WATCH OUT for gluten-free products. Gluten is a natural binder and thickener for foods. When you remove the gluten, you remove the stability of the product. Therefore, this HUGE new market of gluten-free foods are often WORSE than gluten itself. Read the ingredients first and be an informed consumer! It takes some creativity and you might need to spend some time in the kitchen or find a buddy - but it's doable and worth it!

Upgraded Gluten Free Grains (Get Organic Whenever Possible):

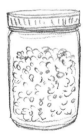

* **Amaranth**
* **Brown Rice**
* **Teff**
* **Millet**
* ***Gluten-Free Oats**
* **Buckwheat**
* **Quinoa**
* **Sorghum**
* ***Steel-cut Oats**

* Oats are Gluten Free. Oats are usually contaminated with other glutenous grains during processing, so wash them first. If you have gluten allergies, look for the gluten-free brands.

Oil

Vegetable oil and Canola oil are **NOT** health foods!

It's soooo upsetting that most of the oils are named vegetable oil because they are nothing but franken-oils. They have been altered beyond recognition in order to create a stability (shelf life) in food and to avoid foods tasting rancid. This creates a bigger profit for the manufactures, and leaves the consumers ingesting more and more toxic ingredients.

Vegetable Oil is EXTREMELY misleading!

These are highly toxic oils and should be avoided:

* Soy / Soybean Oil
* Corn Oil
* Vegetable Oil
* Canola Oil
* Cottonseed Oil
* Sunflower Oil
* Anything with the words Hydrogenated or Modified in it
* **Not a complete list**

According to some research, excessive use of vegetables oils can lead to:

* Asthma
* Blindness
* Heart Disease
* Cancer
* Inflammation
* Serious chronic diseases

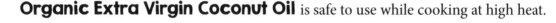

❇ UPGRADED Oils

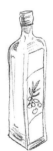

Organic Extra Virgin Coconut Oil is safe to use while cooking at high heat.

After-Cooking Oils:
* Organic Extra Virgin Olive Oil
* Coconut oil is great for any of your oil needs.

You really have to do your research these days with Olive Oil because much of it is cut with other vegetable/canola oils. With Olive Oil, I recommend getting it from a local source and not imported. Some people do well with Organic Sesame Seed oil – test it yourself and see if it works well for you. **The highest quality oils** come in dark-tinted glass bottles, and have the following wording on the label:

* **Expeller-Pressed**
* **Organic**
* **Cold-Pressed**
* **NON-GMO Verified**
* **Minimally Processed**
* **Unrefined**

Fats

REAL Fats are Nourishing. Fake franken-fats are T O X I C. Read the ingredients. **Margarines are fake fake fake**, the fake butters are just that - fake fake fake. **You want Real, Real, Real!** One of the best things you can do for your health is to make sure you are eating quality and nourishing fats.

Toxic Fats

* Hydrogenated or Partially Hydrogenated fats
* Margarine or other fake butter-like substances
* Shortening
* Oils already mentioned (soybean oil, corn oil, etc.)
  NOT a complete list

Because we have been **SOLD** that fats are bad, companies have continued to make low-fat and fat-free frankenfoods that are highly TOXIC for us to consume. They have convinced you that fat is the problem. **Nourishing fats are HEALING**, it's the fake-franken-fats that can be devastating to your health. Even if you are not afraid to consume fats, begin to understand what kinds of fats you consume. Most oils are HIGHLY processed in order to extend shelf life. Take a look at the list below and begin to **incorporate more Nourishing, Energy Fueling and Brain Feeding Upgraded Fats.**

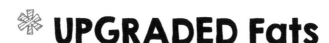

❊ UPGRADED Fats

* **Organic Extra Virgin Coconut Oil**
* **Organic Extra Virgin Olive Oil**
* **Avocados**
* **Organic Nuts and Seeds**
* **Organic Pasture Raised Egg Yolks**
* **Organic Grass Fed Butter or Ghee**
* **Organic Grass Fed Dairy Products** (Includes Goat/Sheep/Cow)
* **Organic Pasture Raised Animal Fat** (Used extensively before the invention of shortening)
* **Not a complete list**

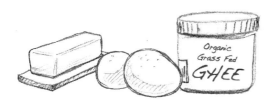
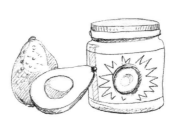
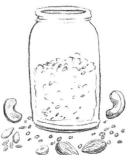

Salt

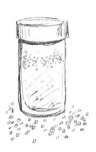

Table Salt is cut with DEXTROSE which is usually derived from GMO corn and the main ingredient in dextrose is refined sugar.
Table salt will also have anti-caking agencies on top of the GMO corn and refined sugar. Refined salt does not have any of the essential nutrients that once graced the salt.

 UPGRADE:
Celtic Sea Salt and Himalayan Salt have trace minerals and essential nutrients in them. Refined salts do NOT.

Food Coloring / Artificial Color

Is a toxic ingredient and unfortunately, this artificial coloring is mostly marketed to kids. Food Coloring has been linked to ADD, ADHD and other Learning Disabilities.

 UPGRADE:
Quality and nourishing foods have beautiful colors naturally; whereas, food colorings are **added to mask** the unappetizing denaturing **color of frankenfoods.**

Artificial Flavorings

Are Toxic, Toxic, TOXIC! In order to taste appealing, these franken-flavors are added to denatured and chemically-processed foods. Artificial flavorings are NEVER needed with real foods.

 UPGRADE:
Nourishing, clean and real foods taste delicious and often a touch of Celtic Sea Salt, fresh herbs, lemon, lime or organic seasonings will naturally bring out flavors.

Natural Flavorings

Unless it says **where** that natural flavor originates, it means that at **one point it was natural**. This is often and unfortunately found in many Organic foods too. According to Dr. Mercola, **MSG, aspartame and bugs in your food are all considered "natural flavors" and "natural colors".** If you REALLY love a food and it says natural flavorings, call the manufacturer and ask them about its origin.

 UPGRADE:
There is an abundance of truly natural flavors in authentically nourishing foods. If you find that the foods you love have chemicals in them and you can't find a version with clean ingredients, consider making your own. See Upgrades and Recipe conversions for more ideas.

MSG

Monosodium Glutamate (MSG) is an excitotoxin that makes food taste really yummy and keeps you coming back for more and more. **MSG is an addictive substance** with a slew of **side effects** that include, but not limited to the following::

* **Headaches**
* **Digestive issues**
* **Skin irritations**

MSG continues to stimulate the appetite, creating a disconnect between the brain and gut so you don't know when you are really full. Think about when you eat a large amount of food at a Chinese restaurant and then feel hungry soon after! MSG is often added to create the umami effect. Umami is that yummy, pleasant, savory, and comforting taste.

Just some of the possible names of MSG:

* Glutamic acid
* Glutamate
* Monosodium glutamate
* Monopotassium glutamate
* Calcium glutamate
* Monoammonium glutamate
* Magnesium glutamate
* Natrium glutamate
* Anything "hydrolyzed"
* Any "hydrolyzed protein"
* Calcium caseinate, Sodium caseinate
* Yeast extract, Torula yeast
* Yeast food, Yeast nutrient
* Autolyzed yeast
* Gelatin
* Textured protein
* Whey protein
* Whey protein concentrate
* Whey protein isolate
* Soy protein
* Soy protein concentrate
* Soy protein isolate
* Anything "protein"
* Anything "protein fortified"
* Soy sauce
* Soy sauce extract
* Anything "enzyme modified"
* Anything containing "enzymes"
* Anything "fermented"
* Anything containing "protease"
* Vetsin
* Ajinomoto
* Umami
* **NOT a complete list**

Visit http://www.truthinlabeling.org/hiddensources.html for more information on MSG.

UPGRADE:

Opt for these alternatives, which naturally bring out the **umami** taste.

* Celtic Sea Salt or Himalayan Salt
* Tomatoes/tomato sauces
* Meats and Fish/Shellfish
* Truffles
* Sweet Potatoes
* Eggs
* Cheese
* Mushrooms
* Organic, NON-GMO Miso Soup
* Seaweed/Nori
* Potatoes
* Carrots
* Coconut Aminos (soy sauce Upgrade)
* Use Organic Whenever Possible

Nuts/Seeds

Many nut and trail mix brands combine an **unhealthy combination of Refined Sugar, Toxic Fats and Table Salt together**. Most nuts and seeds are roasted in toxic oils with added table salt (dextrose/refined sugar).

UPGRADE:

Buy Organic RAW or DRY ROASTED nuts and seeds and create your own trail mix. See sprouting for more ideas on how creating nourishing nut and seed mixes.

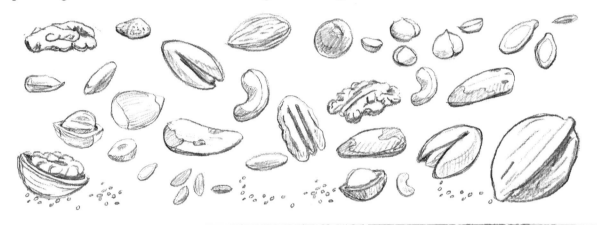

IF you currently eat all or most of the items listed, you might feel overwhelmed. So remember to **take baby steps** and start with the foods that you crave or eat the most.

* **If you crave sugar and sweets a lot, start with Upgraded Sweetener.**

* **If you are a meat and potatoes kind of person, begin by Upgrading your meat to Grass Fed and Pasture Raised.**

* **If you are a processed food lover, seek organic versions.**

* **If you love to cook and fry your food, begin with Upgraded Oils.**

* **If you love dairy and yogurt, begin with Upgraded Dairy products.**

* **If you are a huge soda person, start with an Upgraded Beverage.**

See the Index to find your specific Upgrades or go to page 131 for Upgradeology.

How to Upgrade from Toxic & Artificial Foods

I believe you can eat whatever you want, just as long as the **ingredients** are nourishing and high quality. Get creative in the kitchen and Upgrade where you shop. Begin to read the ingredients on every single item you purchase, and you will slowly begin to understand what chemicals are in the foods you eat. Then refer to Upgrades, (page 131) to find a better solution.

Are you willing to try an experiment? The next time you go to the grocery store, read the ingredients on big brand items that are advertised in magazines and on TV.

1. Look at the front of the package.
Notice the colors, images and any health claims they make.

2. Look at the Nutritional Facts.
This usually backs up what advertisers say on the front of the box.

3. Read EVERY Ingredient.
- Notice how many ingredients there are.

- Notice how many ingredients you really understand.
  For example, are there any real food ingredients or is it a bunch of scientific names?

4. Write down 2-3 suspicious ingredients from this experiment and research them. If you need ideas, look up the ingredients for the following items:

* Baby Formula

* Kid's cereal

* "Healthy" Protein Shake

* "Healthy" Snack Bar

* A Frozen "diet food" Dinner

* Supplemental food for Seniors (i.e. Ensure®)

* Probably anything that you see advertised on a TV commercial

You will probably be horrified at what you find. **Hopefully, after this experiment you will become a committed Ingredient reader.**

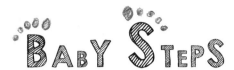

Baby Steps

What item do you feel would best serve you to Upgrade today?

List the possible Upgrades:

Make this Upgrade a new habit and ritual before adding another Upgrade. Tweak and alter this Upgrade until it's satisfying to YOU. Make it taste DELICIOUS! Jot down some possible ways to do that here:

> **Important**: If you don't Upgrade to a food or drink item that you really enjoy, then your choices may feel limited and you are more likely to reach for the ol' toxic gunk again.

In Chapter 4 we discussed:

* The harmful effects of sugar
* The dangers and misleading of food marketing
* Upgraded Sweeteners that are delicious and nutritious
* Symptoms to look for
* What Dr. Weston A. Price discovered
* Just how scary artificial sweeteners truly are
* How to Upgrade from the Toxic and misleading
   Artificial Sweeteners
* How to detox from sugar without biting someone's head off
* How to make your own Stevia
* Variety of ways to Upgrade refined sugar
* Why fruit is an excellent solution to desired sweeteners
* Just some of the MANY names of hidden sugar
* What is really lurking within those frankenfoods

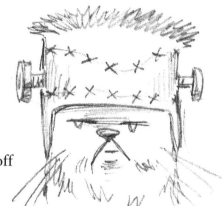

I encourage you to educate yourself about the ingredients in popular foods. Investigate where you find sugar, sugar-free, artificial and diet foods aka frankenfoods. If you want to think clearly and enjoy good health, it's time to return to nature and eat nourishing, REAL, organic foods. There is that old saying *"You are what you eat"*. In reality, **you are what and how you digest and assimilate what you eat.**

Now that you have a better grasp of **REAL vs. toxic/fake ingredients and why it's EXTREMELY important to read ALL food ingredients,** Chapter 5 introduces you to Magic Trio Combinations (Fiber, Protein and Fat). This chapter shows you how to combine foods for optimal blood sugar stabilization. This is essential in the Upgrade process.

I encourage you to do the Baby Steps Exercise at the end of the next chapter, and have fun experimenting with the Recipes. Remember this is NOT an all or nothing program. Do what feels right for YOU! It's like a buffet where you get to choose what to put on your plate and what to leave behind.

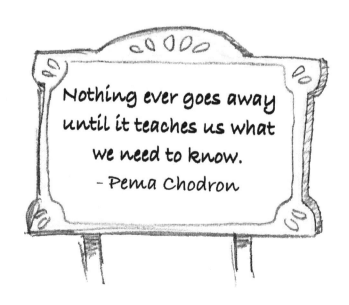

Nothing ever goes away until it teaches us what we need to know.
– Pema Chodron

5 Blood-Sugarology

Food Combinations to Help Harmonize Moods & Stabilize Blood Sugar

Magic Trio Combination

Combining certain foods together is an important step in the Upgrade process.

The Magic Trio Combination is a combination of:

1. **Fiber**
2. **Protein**
3. **Fat**

When you combine Fiber, Protein, and Fat (with spice and/or sauce) **your food cravings stabilize.** Apply endless curiosity…try out different food combos and see if they work for you. If they don't, tweak, adjust, or modify the Magic Trio Combinations until you find the most satisfying fit.

For example, **notice what you crave after eating a piece of fruit.** Then notice what you crave **AFTER eating a piece of fruit with some nut butter, nuts/seeds** or full fat yogurt or raw cheese. Then create your ritual accordingly. Yes, there is the old saying 'fruit alone'. However, with **blood sugar issues** it's important to **slow down fruit (natural sugar) with fat and protein** (i.e. nuts/seeds etc.). This will take the fruit from acting like a fast carb to behaving more like a slow carb (which is what you want).

I have a client who brought an apple to work with her for her mid-day snack. After she ate her apple, she would crave sweets and then visit the candy machine or stop by a coffee shop. Once she began to incorporate a protein and fat with her apple, she no longer craved the candy after eating her apple. She alternated between almond butter and a little baggie of homemade trail mix of dry roasted nuts and seeds, and added her own Celtic Sea Salt. Her snack includes Fiber, Protein and Fat. Thus, her snack is more satisfying, sustained her longer throughout the day, and kept her away from the candy bars.

Winning Magic Trio Combinations

Review a recipe and note if it contains **Fiber, Protein**, and **Fat. Some foods include all three such as:**

* Avocados
* Ground flax seeds
* Chia seeds
* Nuts/Seeds

So if you have an Avocado, your Protein, Fiber, and Fat are taken care of in one meal or snack! Just add a little Celtic Sea Salt and it's delish!

Here's a simple recipe that uses this winning combination:

Fiber: Asparagus and garlic
Protein: Pecans and asparagus (remember, most vegetables have protein!)
Fat/Sauce: Pecans, coconut oil
Spices: Lemon, Celtic Sea Salt

Creamy Asparagus Soup

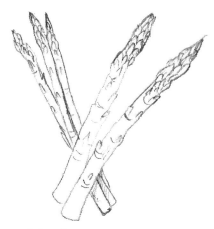

* 10 thick or 25 thin or 1 bunch of organic asparagus – steamed/boiled
* 2/3 cup organic pecans
* 2 cups purified water
* 2 TBSP organic coconut oil
* 3 TBSP organic lemon juice (freshly squeezed)
* 2 cloves organic garlic
* ½ tsp Celtic Sea Salt

Directions:

1. Steam or lightly boil asparagus. For thick asparagus, approx. 10 minutes and for thin asparagus, approx. 5 minutes.
2. Let asparagus cool and then blend with 2 cups of water (use water you used to cook the asparagus).
3. In blender: place asparagus, 2 cups cooking water, pecans, olive oil, lemon juice, garlic and salt.
4. Blend until desired consistency is reached.
5. Serve warm and garnish with cilantro.

Try these Magic Trio Combinations for yourself:

*Vegetables are mostly fiber (and nutrients) and they also contain protein!
Use ORGANICS Whenever Possible!

What Foods Fall into Each Category?

Nutrient FIBER	Quality PROTEIN	Nourishing FATS
Vegetables	Vegetables	Organic Extra Virgin Coconut Oil
Fruit	Nuts	Organic Extra Virgin Olive Oil
Nuts	Seeds	Organic Nuts/Seeds
Seeds	Beans/Legumes	Organic Avocado
Whole Grains	Grains	
Beans/ Legumes		
	Pasture Raised, Hormone and Anti-biotic free Animal Products Such As Dairy/Eggs/Meat/Fish	Organic Butter or Ghee Organic Pasture Raised Egg Yolks

*The Magic Trio Combinations listed above are not a complete list

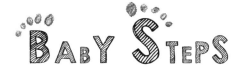

Snack ONE

Pick a time today and tomorrow that you can do this experiment.

1. Have a piece of fruit for your snack. Eat this at least 2 hours after a meal and at least 1 hour before another meal or snack.

2. After eating it, notice how long you feel satisfied.

   Do you immediately want something else?

   Does it create more cravings?

   If so, what do you crave?

3. Write down how you feel right after eating the fruit:

   Set a timer and write down how you feel after 30 minutes:

   After 1 hour:

   After 1.5 hours:

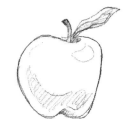

Snack TWO

1. Have a piece of fruit with either nut butter or some raw or dry roasted nuts/seeds, or another Upgraded protein/fat that you enjoy.

2. Write down how you feel right after eating it:

   Then write down how you feel after 30 minutes:

   After 1 hour:

   After 1.5 hours:

Which snack satisfied you longer?

1. Compare your Snack #1 and Snack #2 notes.

2. Which snack satisfied you the longest?

3. Did Snack #2 keep you from immediate cravings?

4. Other observations?

   Once you've completed this little experiment, you will know the snack combinations that serve you best in the long run. Do what works best for you!

Fiber, Protein, and Fat at Every Meal and Snack = Blood Sugar Stabilization

These foods fall into many categories (see below). Pay attention to the categories that contain all three. This makes it easier to include your Fiber, Protein, and Fat at every meal.

Simple foods that include the Magic Trio Combination:

* Avocado
* Chia Seeds
* Ground Flax Seeds
* Hemp Seeds
* Nuts/Seeds, Nut Butters

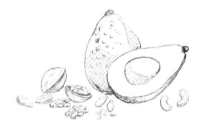

These are also very portable! Experiment with your own Magic Trio Combinations to meet the needs of your taste buds and cravings.

Easily create your Magic Trio Combination by ADDING a small amount of Nourishing Fat to:

* Fruits
* Vegetables
* Beans
* Legumes
* Whole Grains

Fiber, Protein, and Fat Chart (not a complete list)

Adding a little spice or Celtic Sea Salt to your food will naturally bring out the flavors and make them more delicious. **Use ORGANIC Whenever Possible! Note:** the top part of the chart is plant-based and useful for every food plan.

FIBER	PROTEIN	FATS	Spice
Vegetables	Vegetables	Extra Virgin Coconut Oil	Celtic Sea Salt
Nuts/Seeds	Nuts	Extra Virgin Olive Oil	Pepper
Beans/Legumes	Seeds	Nuts	Cinnamon
Whole Grains	Beans	Seeds	Paprika
Fresh Fruit	Legumes	Nut Butters	Cayenne
Sprouts	Whole Grains (i.e. Quinoa)	Cacao Butter	Coriander
Chia Seeds	**Chia Seeds**	**Chia Seeds**	Cardamom
Ground Flax Seeds	**Ground Flax Seeds**	**Ground Flax Seeds**	Garlic
Avocado	**Avocado**	**Avocado**	Ginger
	Pasture Raised, Hormone and Anti-biotic free Animal Products Such As Dairy/Eggs/Meat/Fish	Grass-Fed Butter or Ghee Pasture Raised Egg Yolks	

Create your own chart with foods that you enjoy, remember that most foods will fall into more than one category:

FIBER	PROTEIN	FATS	Spice

Condiments

Upgrade your condiments! Most condiments are full of sugar, toxic oils, table salt, etc. Ideally, find organic brands with simple, quality ingredients. If you can't find a nourishing Upgrade, begin experimenting by altering recipes and making your own.

Beware of hidden sugars. Did you know that most Balsamic Vinegars have refined sugar in them? Instead, use Apple Cider Vinegar and/or Coconut Vinegar. Once again, remember to always read ingredients. Regular vinegar can easily turn into sugar in your body. If you are sensitive to sugar, it's important to be aware of anything with alcohol or vinegar in it.

Basic condiments to Upgrade:

Most store bought condiments have refined and/or artificial sugar and MSG in them.
* Mayonnaise (sugar, vinegar, toxic oils)
* Mustard (sugar, white vinegar)
* Ketchup (sugar, white vinegar)
* Soy Sauce (soy, sugar, MSG)
* Sweet and Sour Sauces (sugar, artificial ingredients)
* BBQ Sauces (sugar, artificial ingredients)
* Table Salt (dextrose/sugar and anti-caking agencies, stripped of nutrients)
* Hot Sauces (sugar, vinegar, often msg)

Upgrade to **nourishing ingredients**, learn to make your own **sauces** (pages 108, 138-141).

It's all about the SAUCE!

If you think about it, **what really makes a food taste good?** It's all about **the sauce!** With a sauce, you add texture and flavor - it's what makes the dish delish!

Many highly processed foods have a base which is something they have to boil the heck out of to eliminate harmful bacteria. The food-like-substance is then bleached (to take out the unappealing color), and then artificial flavor, color and texture are added in to make it appear like food again. Whatever processed snack foods you eat, it's not the actual thing (like the grain, potato, or corn inside them) you are tasting. It's really the spice and sauce that makes them taste good.

Try this experiment. Take some sliced carrots (or any vegetable you enjoy), put them in your favorite processed chip or snack bag, smear them around in the spice or sauce, and then see how good they taste. **Most processed or packaged foods have a large quantity of ingredients in them**. However, it's not the base that you taste, it's the sauce! Processed foods are heated and devoid of any taste or flavor because it's the cheapest stuff used. Just like fruit juices...do you really think that food manufacturers use fresh, vibrant organic fruits in their bottled juices? No, they use the rejects and they have to heat and then flavor them so that:

1. It tastes the same every single time
2. It has a long shelf life and
3. It looks appealing – thanks to artificial coloring, flavoring, and each manufacturers 'secret sauce'.

If you think about it...ALL processed foods taste the same... every... single... time. Why? Because a chemical formula was created to keep that consistency. Have you ever had a fresh batch of organic berries? Notice how some taste sweeter while others taste tarter? Each berry in the batch tastes slightly different. Just as identical twins are not 100% identical. There is always something unique about everybody, which includes every NATURAL piece of food.

Let's get back to the sauce. The focus here is your taste buds and the sauce. **You have to find OR create a sauce that tastes DELICIOUS to you, otherwise you may nose-dive right back into the artificial stuff.**

Ever had a really good salad? Maybe a Caesar salad that was drenched in dressing and croûtons that were smothered in seasonings? When you learn to season, spice and sauce your food to your liking, then you have the golden ticket to feeling satisfied with your food. It's all about the texture and sauce. Create foods in the texture you prefer: i.e. crispy and crunchy, mushy, al dente, etc. Learn to prepare basic items such as a big salad, steamed vegetables, cooked rice or beans, or a tender piece of protein. Then spend the majority of your time creating a delicious sauce. Next up, tasty Sauce recipes!

It's all about the SAUCE!

When Upgrading your Sauce:

* **Purchase an Organic version with the cleanest Ingredients!**

* **Learn to make your own.** (See next page and pages 138-141)

Worcestershire-ish Sauce*

* 1/2 cup Organic Raw Apple Cider Vinegar
* 2 TBSP Organic Tamarind
* 2 TBSP Raw Honey
* 1 TBSP Organic Blackstrap Molasses
* 1 Lime (juiced)
* 1/2 tsp ground Clove
* 1/2 tsp Onion powder
* 1/4 tsp Garlic
* 1/4 tsp Cayenne or Chili Powder

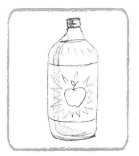

Directions:

Mix all ingredients together in a shaker bottle or in a recycled dressing bottle.

This won't taste exactly like the Worcestershire sauce you knew before, but give it a whirl and add your own flair to it.

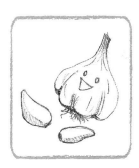

*Inspired by: www.foodrenegade.com

Hollandaise Sauce*

* 1/2 cup Organic Grass Fed Butter, Ghee, Avocado **OR** Coconut Oil
* 3 Organic Pasture Raised egg yolks or Flax Egg Alternative (page 231)
* 2 TBSP Lemon juice (freshly squeezed)
* Celtic Sea Salt to taste
* Pinch of Cayenne pepper (optional)

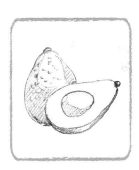

Directions:

1. Gently melt the butter over medium heat on stove.

2. In a blender, combine yolks, lemon juice, sea salt, and cayenne (optional).

3. Blend on medium or puree speed for about 30 seconds.

4. Slowly add butter, and continue to blend on medium or puree speed until desired consistency.

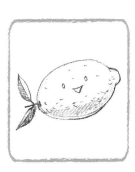

*Inspired by: www.motherearthnews.com/real-food/how-to-make-hollandaise-sauce-zmrz12amzhir.aspx

How to Create Your Own Sauces & Spreads*

* First - Choose One Item For **The Base**

* Cooked and mashed beans (any bean such as kidney, chickpea, mung, black, etc.)
* Cooked and blended whole grain (such as brown or basmati rice, quinoa, etc.)
* Blended, cooked vegetables (root vegetables such as carrots and celeriac work well)
* Soup Broth or Water

* Second - Choose from the following tastes and textures

Sweet

Any Upgraded Sweetener
(Pages 77, 83-85)
Stevia
Coconut Sugar
Coconut Nectar
RAW Honey
Brown Rice Syrup
Yacon

Sour or Zesty

Apple Cider Vinegar
Lemon or Lime juice
Organic mustard
Sauerkraut
Tomato
Garlic
Ginger
Onion

Salty

Celtic Sea Salt
Himalayan Salt
Miso
Soy sauce
Coconut Aminos
Sauerkraut
Celery
Dulse or Seaweed Flakes

* Third - Choose a thickener if needed

* **Arrowroot powder:** Use instead of cornstarch.

* **Kuzu:** Excellent for thickening soups and stews.

* **Agar Agar:** Creates a gel-like substance. Excellent for creating a custard, gelatin or pudding-like texture.

* **Avocado:** Creates a pudding, cream or mayonnaise-like substance.

* **Ground Chia Seeds:** Creates a gel-like substance for pudding or egg replacement.

* **Ground Flax Seeds:** Creates a gel-like substance for egg replacement.

* **Coconut Oil or Coconut Butter:** Use instead of other oils or dairy for a creamy texture.

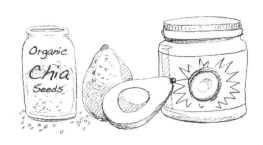

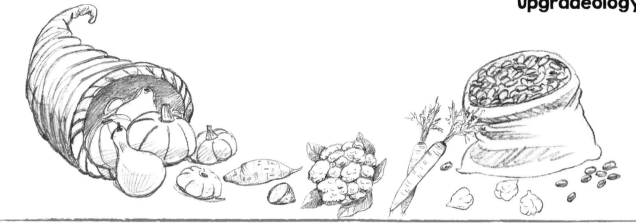

Nutty

Tahini
Almond butter
Cashews
Brazil Nuts
Sunflower Seeds
Hemp Seeds
Toasted nuts or seeds

Refreshing

Green onion
Lemon peel
Caraway seed
Dill
Thyme
Marjoram
Parsley
Cilantro

Creamy

Avocado
Olive Oil
Coconut Oil
Coconut Butter
Plain Grass Fed Yogurt
Pasture Raised Egg Yolk

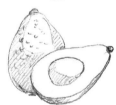

❋ Fourth - Combine desired ingredients into a food processor or blender and create your desired taste and texture.

If TOO Thick:

1. Start with your base and add 1 TBSP water to thin sauce.

2. Slowly add more water/liquids and flavors.

3. Taste as you go to make it just right.

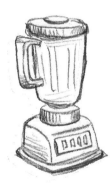

More 'make-it-yourself' ideas on pages 138-141.
Explore, play, create and use organic whenever possible!

*   Inspired by: *The Self-Healing Cookbook: Whole Foods To Balance Body, Mind and Moods* by Kristina Turner

Release the Diet Mentality

Release that diet mentality when thinking about transitioning to nourishing foods. Beware of getting stingy with the sauce, and resist the urge to start counting calories. Be very, very generous with the sauce. Include nourishing fats and spices in your sauce. These alone can help you love and enjoy your Upgraded foods.

Nourishing foods are the place to indulge. The reason you can't control yourself with unhealthy food is that it's FULL of flavor enhancers. For example, MSG is a chemical that triggers your brain to want MORE. MSG also turns off your fullness sensor and turns on your need for more, more, AND more. Another trigger can be the combination of sugar, fat and salt. Did you ever eat something and continued eating it even though you felt full? If you look at the ingredients, I'm fairly certain you would find either MSG and/or sugar which keeps you coming back for more and more (along with the key binge effects of refined sugar, fat and salt).

Notice a bag of chips. Do you usually finish the entire bag? If it's a big bag, you may eat until you are sick. If it's a small bag, you may lick out every last crumb. It really comes down to the ingredients inside that bag/package that creates your cravings.

Eating quality food is easier than it seems. Find fresh fruits and vegetables that appeal to you and then get creative with sauces, dips, spices, and variety. Find natural food stores or farmers markets in town that sell nourishing organic produce and organic packaged foods (read the ingredients). Watch out for hidden sugars and artificial ingredients. Find foods that you enjoy and satisfy you. Avocados, nuts and seeds, and homemade granola bars or trail mixes (see recipe section on page 230) make hearty and portable snacks.

❓ **What are your belief's about diets?**

❓ **Write down a few of your diet experiences and why you didn't stay on that diet?**

❓ **What new belief would assist you in a more consistent healthy food plan, rather than the ping-pong dieting?**

Nourishing Fats

As mentioned in Chapter 4, if you're concerned about cholesterol that is found in animal products, use more plant-based fats in your meals (not the fake butters/margarines/low/non-fat items). **When it comes to cholesterol, the real issue is fake fats, chemical processing, and toxic oils.** The quality/natural fats are GOOD cholesterol that your body needs and wants. The fake and toxic fats the ones that create dis-harmony in your system. Bottom line, don't fear the quality fats!

Plant-Based Nourishing FATS

* Avocados - no cholesterol and no sodium (also great for baby foods)
* Coconut Oil & Butter - no cholesterol and no sodium
* Cacao Butter & Nibs - contain magnesium and antioxidants
* Organic Extra Virgin Olive Oil
* Organic Olives
* Nuts & Seeds
    * Walnuts
    * Brazil Nuts
    * Hemp Seeds
    * Chia Seeds
    * Sunflower Seeds
    * Almonds
    * Not a complete list

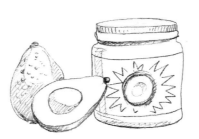
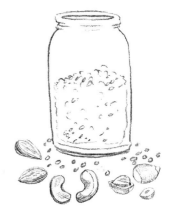

Nourishing Animal FATS

* Organic Pasture Raised Unsalted Butter
* Organic Ghee
* Pasture Raised Eggs
* Pasture Raised Lard, Suet, Duck Fat, etc.
* Organic Raw Dairy/Cheese (Goat, Sheep, Cow)
* Full Fat Protein - not the lean stuff (i.e. chicken: the dark meat has MORE nutrients than the light meat)

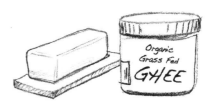

Old	Upgrade
Canola Oil	Olive Oil, Coconut Oil, Ghee, Animal Fat or Butter
Vegetable Oil	Olive Oil, Coconut Oil, Ghee, Animal Fat or Butter
Fried Food Oil	Coconut Oil or Animal Fat/Ghee/Butter
Spray Oil (such as Pam®)	Light coating of Coconut Oil or Animal Fat/Butter You can get a pump canister that will work with liquid oil. This can be tricky in cold weather if the fat becomes solid.

Breakfast

What's the most important meal of the day? (Hint: breakfast) That's right, it's breakfast! And why is it so important? Blood sugar stabilization!

Trouble starts when you skip breakfast. I had a tendency to skip breakfast so I know how tough it can be if you are not a breakfast person. However, once I embraced breakfast early in the morning, something magical happened. I stopped overeating and binge eating at night! Many of my clients also struggle with eating breakfast. I've heard it all -- I'm too busy in the morning, I'm not hungry in the morning, or I don't have time to make breakfast. I've included Breakfast Upgrades to make it simple and easy for you. Once you embrace breakfast and start to experience the benefits, you'll wonder why you fought against eating breakfast for so long.

If you have an extremely busy morning, try some of these easy breakfast ideas:

* Make a smoothie the night before and place in refrigerator to grab and go in the morning.

* If you like eggs, make a frittata that will last a few days.

* Add chia seeds in some almond milk the night before. This makes a great porridge for the following morning.

  See Recipe section (starting page 230) for more breakfast ideas.

Many of these breakfast items can be quickly whipped together and then grab and go. Your "Gotta Go Bag" (page 118) makes it quick and easy for you (see Snacks next) and is a good replacement for any meal or snack you miss. Carry chia seeds and your favorite Upgraded Sweetener in your "Gotta Go Bag" for a quick, healthy pick-me-up.

If you are already a committed breakfast person, fantastic! Keep with it and see if your breakfast needs an Upgrade. If you eat the same breakfast every day, then this experiment may be a stretch for you, but it's worth it...why? Different foods create different reactions. If you are too busy during the week to try something new, no problem! Dedicate time to experiment during the weekend.

Be sure to write down what you eat in your Food/Mood Journal and how you feel after breakfast. Refer to Journal at end of this chapter. I've had many clients find the kick start to their day because of breakfast and their Food/Mood Journal. After eating, notice how your energy level feels, what kind of mood do you experience, and how does your body and digestive track feel?

* How do you feel right after eating?

* How do you feel two hours later?

After completing this exercise, you may discover that you are sensitive to certain foods. A food sensitivity or allergy may be your body's way of telling you what food is more appropriate for your body's needs and current lifestyle.

Write out at least three different breakfast options so you have variety. I have many clients who like to eat the same thing every morning. It's helpful for your body to have a little variety. It also helps to notice what foods digest well and what foods do not. If you eat the same thing every day and experience the same symptoms every day (i.e. bloating, fatigue, headaches, moodiness etc.) then how do you know where these symptoms originate?

To be successful with your breakfast investigations, think about how you will plan and prepare your breakfast for three days. List the food items you will need for at least three different breakfasts in the upcoming week. If you have a busy day ahead of you (and value sleep over food), prepare your breakfast foods in the evening so you have an easier grab and go morning.

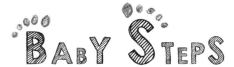

 Start with breakfast in mind. If you plan just one nourishing meal a day, let it be breakfast. Write down some breakfast ideas that appeal to you:

 If you have a busy morning, make a little time in the evening to prepare snacks for the next day so you can just grab and go. What is your plan for snacks:

 As you get into the rhythm of planning ahead, create a menu the day before based on what you have on hand for meals and snacks. Start with at least one homemade or Upgraded meal or snack per day and build from there:

Snacks & Blood Sugar Stabilization

Nourishing snacks, in combination with breakfast, keep your blood sugar stable. Snacks also give you consistent energy throughout the day. If you get the mid-day slumps, then remember to snack. If you know your slump is at 3:30 pm every day, set a timer for 3 pm and eat your snack at 3 pm (or sooner). Experiment with eating a meal or snack EVERY 2-3 hours, especially if you have blood sugar issues.

Blood sugar issues seem to be the norm these days. They do not just affect diabetics or people with hypoglycemia. Certain foods, and stimulants such as caffeine, go through your blood stream quicker. Caffeine can give you a huge rise (why so many people feel that they MUST have coffee to get going in the morning. For those hooked on caffeine, it also acts as an appetite suppressant (see Caffeine section on page 144) which disrupts your blood sugar balance.

When blood sugars get too low, you become cranky, easily frustrated, shaky, light headed, and don't make the wisest decisions. **Remember this:** Don't make any important decisions on an empty stomach. Why? Because your brain does not have the proper balancing fuel it needs when your blood sugar drops too low.

1. **STABLE** blood sugar graph (below).
   Starting the day with a nourishing breakfast and then having snacks and meals throughout the day. Drinking purified water and incorporating the Magic Trio Combination into meals and snacks.

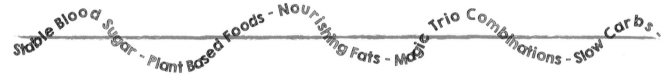

2. **UNSTABLE** blood sugar graph (below).
   Starting the day without breakfast or beginning with coffee and a refined sweet or processed food or cereal will give you that initial BOOST of energy you are looking for and then DROP you down low. Once you realize it, you may go for the quickest energy source available, more caffeine and refined sugars/processed foods. You have highs and lows of energy throughout the day.

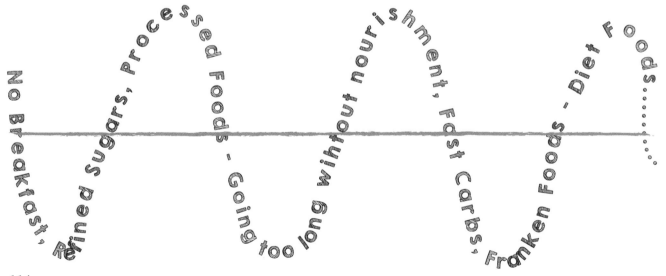

Once you are able to **Upgrade** the items you love, incorporate the **Magic Trio Combinations** and eat at more consistent times. You will notice a **Natural Rise** in your **ENERGY**. This is the energy you have sought through caffinated drinks and refined foods. The **Easier** and **QUICKER** route to **Sustained Energy** and **Stable Blood Sugar** is through **Nourishing Foods** and the **Magic Trio Combinations**.

Energizing snack "pick-me-ups" to eat throughout your day:

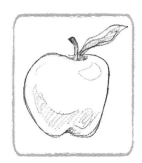

* Homemade granola bars or trail mix (see recipes).

* Avocado with a pinch of Celtic Sea Salt.

* Chia seeds in water with Goji berries and organic coconut sugar or organic green leaf stevia.

* Combination of Fresh fruit and nuts or nut butters - i.e. apple with almond butter or fresh berries with a handful of almonds and sunflower seeds Organic full fat Yogurt (cow/goat/sheep) with organic fresh ground flax seeds OR chia seeds.
  Note: Chia seeds can be whole or ground - however you like them. Flax seeds are ideally ground or sprouted for digestibility. You can also get organic flax seed oil (never heat flax seed oil).

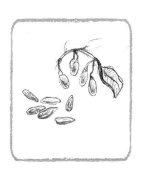

* Make your own chia pods with chia seeds, almond milk, cinnamon, ginger, cardamom, coconut sugar and whatever else you desire!

* Organic unsweetened chocolate with some nuts, seeds and raw honey.

* Organic gluten free granola.

* Celery, avocado, sunflower seeds, and sea salt - I love this one because it's like a mock tuna.

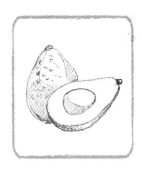

* Organic sliced veggies and organic hummus.

* If you like crunch, go for crunchy veggies such as carrots, jicama, celery, or other root veggies. I also LOVE sugar snap peas, but they are seasonal. Stock up on sugar snap peas during the summer. Dip them in guacamole, almond butter, or hummus. Find your favorite Upgraded sauce or dip and keep a lot of it on hand. Notice the everyday snacks you eat and see how you can Upgrade them!

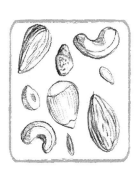

Note: about dried fruit - most have refined sugar, sulfur and possibly other ingredients in them. Read your ingredients! The best dried fruits are organic dates or goji berries. Other nourishing options: organic raisins, dried apricots, or figs.

See recipe section on page 230 and get organic whenever possible.

Fast Carbs / Slow Carbs & Fruit Carbs

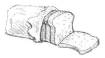

Fast Carbs

Nourishing carbohydrates are NOT the enemy. It's the toxic, chemically-processed ingredients that harm you. Carbohydrates are essential and nourishing; they break down into natural sugar to fuel your body (unlike refined sugar). You need carbohydrates for fuel, but not in the quantity or toxicity in which they are consumed these days. The difference between fast carbs and slow carbs is how quickly your body breaks down these foods into sugar for energy. Slow and steady is what your body thrives on!

If you want potato chips, make them yourself or find a brand made with coconut oil. Craving bread? Find an organic sprouted brand with the cleanest ingredients or make a homemade sourdough or gluten-free bread. There are tons of recipes out there with nutritious ingredients that will satisfy every palate. See Upgrades on page 131 for more ideas.

When craving 'fast carbs' such as sweet foods, refined and processed meals and snacks, coffee and/or energy drinks, it's really your body calling out for energy. These fast carbs actually zap your energy and take your blood sugar on a roller coaster ride. When you crave those fast carbs, begin to see if there are any 'fruit carbs' or 'slow carbs' that would satisfy you instead. If not, begin to Upgrade those fast carbs into more nourishing foods so that they give you energy instead of steal it from you.

Fast Carbs to Upgrade

Foods with a high glycemic index, including processed carbohydrates such as breads, cereals, most desserts, and sugar are considered fast carbs. The carbohydrate molecules found in these foods are smaller, especially in the case of sugar, and are broken down rapidly into sugars in your intestines. If eaten regularly, fast carbs keep your blood sugar elevated. They also contribute to obesity, Type 2 Diabetes, metabolic disturbances, and cardiovascular disease. These are the carbs to Upgrade!

What are some of your favorite FAST Carbs?

What can you use as an alternative to the FAST Carbs you listed above?

See Upgrades on page 131.

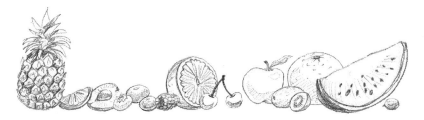

Fruit Carbs

Most fruits are high glycemic (except lemon, lime, berries and grapefruit) and are also considered fast carbs. Fruits can be a nourishing 'fast carb', especially if they are combined with a protein and fat to slow them down. In order to avoid confusion, let's call these 'fruit carbs'.

What is your favorite 'Fruit Carb'?

What protein and fiber can you add to your 'Fruit Carb' to take it from a fast fruit carb to a slow fruit carb?

Slow Carbs

Slow carbs contain fiber and protein (whole grains) and sometimes fat (nuts/seeds). These components slow down the food's conversion to glucose in your bloodstream. Slow carbs provide your body with energy over an extended period of time without a rapid drop in blood sugar. Slow carbs have a more complicated molecular chain which is why they are also called complex carbohydrates.

Foods with a low glycemic index are considered SLOW carbs:

* Vegetables
* Whole Grains
* Nuts/Seeds
* Beans/Legumes

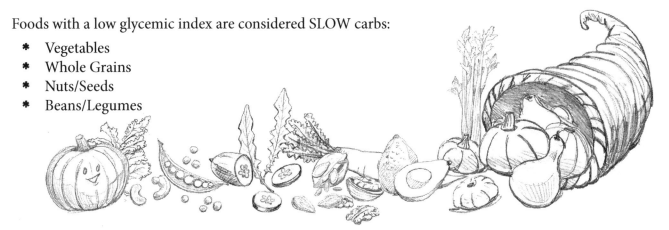

Upgrade to SLOW carbs throughout your day to keep blood sugar stable.

List some SLOW carbs you eat:

What are some SLOW carbs that you want to eat more of and/or experiment with?

Recap

* **Fast Carbs** - (processed/refined grains and sugar) – **Research Upgrade options.**

* **Fruit Carbs – Excellent sources of energy** – need to be slowed down with with an added protein and fat.

* **Slow Carbs – Excellent sources of sustained nourishment and energy.**

"Gotta Go Bag"

The "Gotta Go Bag" has been the saving grace for me and many of my clients. For example, a client really struggled with eating healthy at work. Despite eating a nourishing breakfast and lunch, she still couldn't resist the processed and refined treats that her co-workers brought into the office. The temptation was even greater for her, because she didn't bring snacks with her and always felt hungry throughout the day. Not to mention, there weren't any healthy food choices available nearby.

How did she accomplish her Snack Upgrade? We chose her Upgrades based on her favorite snacks foods, and created a "Gotta Go Bag" for her – a simple way to bring nourishing snacks with her to work. For her, it was homemade trail mix. As a result, her Upgrades were a big success! When we talked two weeks later, she mentioned she only ate the unhealthy office treats ONCE… because she forgot her snacks that day. She loves the taste of her snacks and commented that they were both delicious and satisfying. Another helpful tip (so she didn't feel hungry or feel tempted throughout her work day): she ate an Upgraded snack or sipped a smoothie every two hours. Now she feels like she has more 'willpower' and doesn't feel as tempted like she did in the past – thanks to her "Gotta Go Bag" and snacks!

There is a good reason why my client immediately reached for the office treats during her work day. She was hungry, her blood sugar was low, AND there were tempting foods around. If you are prepared with Upgraded food and snacks (and when you feel nourished by them), then it becomes easier to focus on your own food and you will begin to pass by the temptations.

Items to Include in YOUR 'Gotta Go Bag'

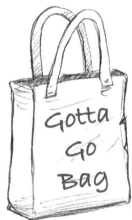

* _____
* _____
* _____
* _____
* _____
* _____
* _____

Make your "Gotta Go Bag" fit your personal lifestyle AND your taste buds. It can be as simple as little bags of chia seeds and a bottle of water. It can be as complex as nuts, seeds, nut butters, and pre-made, homemade protein shakes, packed meals, etc. It can be a cooler with extra snacks or whatever suits your needs and lifestyle.

In your "Gotta Go Bag", include non-perishable snacks that you LOVE and will SATISFY you on the fly. **With preparation, the foods inside your "Gotta Go Bag" help you stay clear, focused and on the Upgraded path. When you are hungry, this is the PERFECT time for advertisers to sway you to buy what THEY want you to eat.** When you are hungry and feel unsatisfied, that's when you give into that candy or sweet, or your car automatically steers you to the drive-thru. Being unprepared, tired, stressed or overly hungry has more to do with the inability to stick to a nourishing food plan than almost anything else.

1. **Be prepared and always have extra food and water with you.**

2. **Your food needs to be flavorful and tasty so that you look forward to eating it.**

You can carry around your "Gotta Go Bag" all week long, but if other people's food always seems more attractive than your food, you may find your food moldy in the trunk of your car a year from now.

Even if your snacks don't seem like the perfect Upgrade, **even the smallest Upgrade IS progress** and helps move you closer to long-term health goals.

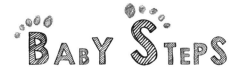

 Find an Upgraded snack that you REALLY enjoy and bring it along with you to work, school, activities, etc.

 Keep track of how long it's been since you ate and begin to incorporate snacks. Eat a snack or meal every 2-3 hours. Notice your blood sugar levels (i.e. your mood and energy). Do you feel light headed? Do you instantly become irritated or agitated? Do you reach a point where you suddenly feel starving? Are you sluggish and NEED that caffeine pick-me-up?

 Make your own "Gotta Go Bag". Keep snacks and back-ups with you. These snack Upgrades help you ENJOY THE TASTE OF your food and keep you away from the low blood sugar danger zone.

Enzymes

Eating begins with the simple act of chewing. Chewing leads to smooth digestion and greater assimilation of nutrients by initiating the release of digestive enzymes that break down food. Do you eat nourishing foods but still struggle with digestive issues? It may be time to introduce digestive enzymes to your belly. Our bodies have two sources for enzymes. The digestive system naturally produces enzymes and raw foods provide additional enzymes needed for digestion. Sometimes as you age, your body stops producing much-needed enzymes. Eating processed foods that are devoid of necessary enzymes can exacerbate a lack of digestive enzymes. Stress also affects your body's ability to produce digestive enzymes.

Enzymes that help digest your food:

* Amylase Enzymes are responsible for digesting carbohydrates, starches and sugars. Examples: Lactase breaks down the lactose found in milk. Sucrose digests complex sugars and starches.
* Protease Enzymes are primarily responsible for breaking down the proteins found in meat, nuts, and eggs. For example, peptidase breaks down everything from peptide proteins to amino acids.
* Lipase Enzymes are responsible for breaking down fats. They digest the fat in nuts, oils, meats, and dairy products.
* Cellulase Enzymes are responsible for digesting cellulose or plant fibers. These are essential enzymes.

When you eat a large meal and feel sleepy afterwards, it's a sign that your body is working overtime to digest your food. If you eat nourishing foods and still struggle with digestive issues, your body may not produce enough digestive enzymes. It makes sense to add more whole, raw foods into your meals and snacks to help increase digestive enzymes. This is not always the best option for everyone, because some people have difficulty digesting raw foods. This can be addressed by taking supplemental digestive enzymes with meals and snacks.

By taking a high quality digestive enzyme with your meals, you may be able to ease some of the following issues:

* Do you feel gassy and bloated after eating?

* Do you get full quickly?

* After a bowel movement, do you see undigested food in the toilet?

* Does your stool look oily (undigested fat)?

Benefits of supplemental enzymes:

* Calms upset digestive systems
* Increases nutrients absorbed from food
* Increased mental and physical performance
* Replaces some of the enzymes you use. The supply of enzymes your body has must be constantly renewed
* Enzymes interact with hormones to control bodily functions
* Triggers vitamin absorption
* Helps to digest proteins, fats, and carbohydrates
* Reduces inflammation and joint pain
* Clears the digestive track of parasites and yeast

If you don't want to take a supplement, add high enzymatic foods to your meals. In order to benefit from enzymatic properties, these foods need to be organic and RAW (see list below). Heat ranging from 104-115 degrees and up will destroy enzyme benefits.

Excellent enzymatic foods to try:

* **Papayas** contain the enzyme papain and help break down proteins.

* **Pineapples** contain the enzyme bromelain which helps break down proteins and decrease inflammation. The greatest amount of bromelain is found in the stem, but the stem is hard to eat.

* **Sprouts** have 100 times more enzymes than fruits and vegetables. They have a ton of nutrients and assist with better digestion.

* **Raw and SPROUTED Nuts and Seeds** contain the enzyme lipase. Sprouting nuts and seeds are excellent because they break down enzyme inhibitors which naturally occur in raw nuts and seeds to protect them from going rancid. Sprouting releases the inhibitors to allow enzymes to be digestible. To sprout nuts and seeds, see chart on page 184.

* **Raw Fruits and Vegetables** contain the enzyme amylase. This is great for breaking down carbohydrates! Again, do not cook fruits and veggies if you want the full benefit of enzymes!

If you eat plenty of nutritious, organic raw foods but still experience symptoms, consider taking a supplemental enzyme to help ease these symptoms. Regardless of where you get your enzymes (from food or supplements), they are completely essential for digestion. You can also find digestive enzyme supplement information on my website: www.Upgradeology.com or www.NicoleWhiteWellness.com.

Note: be sure to read the ingredients for the supplements you purchase. There are many unnecessary binders and fillers in most of the store bought supplements. With digestive enzymes you want to make sure you are getting them from a quality source.

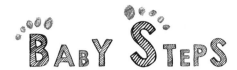

 Notice how much or how little you chew your food.

 Bring awareness while eating your food. Begin to chew your food a few MORE times than normal. If you have any digestive issues, begin to chew your food even MORE.

 Slow down your eating. Put down your utensil after each bite and notice the taste and texture of your food as you eat it. Most of us eat while multi-tasking and are unaware of the food we eat.

Probiotic Foods

Your digestive tract has TRILLIONS of bacteria in it. Positive bacteria in your gut keeps your immune system healthy and helps you assimilate your food. Bacteria are essential for good digestive health, but sometimes things get a bit out of whack in your body. For example, antibiotics get rid of the good gut bacteria along with the 'bad' bacteria or infection. This can lead to symptoms such as diarrhea, eczema, intolerance to foods, allergies, weakened immune symptoms, and a host of other ailments.

Fortunately, there are several ways you can renew and replenish the beneficial bacteria in your gut. Probiotic foods have been reported to help with diarrhea, Crohn's disease, irritable bowel syndrome, and treat yeast infections (Candida). When you eat probiotic foods, you introduce new, beneficial bacteria into your digestive system. The new bacteria join others in the gut to aid with digestion, healing the body, and building upon the positive gut flora. When using food as medicine, get clean reliable sources (including your probiotics)!

There are a wide variety of probiotic-rich, fermented foods that you can buy or make. Sauerkraut, fermented cabbage, has a ton of live cultures (see recipe on page 124)! There's also evidence that it can help with allergies. It's packed full of fiber, vitamins, and nutrients!

Upgrade by adding one of the following foods into your daily menu:

Kefir

Kefir is fermented milk (goat, sheep or cow). Kefir can also be made using coconut milk (vegan). Kefir contains numerous beneficial bacteria. Try to find an organic version. You can easily make your own kefir with fresh raw goat/sheep, cow milk, or coconut water and a kefir starter grain (found in the dairy section in many natural grocery stores/health food stores).

Kombucha

Kombucha is a fermented beverage. It is centuries old and packed with healing gut bacteria. Some brands are better than others. Small batch distributors may be better than mass market ones. You can also make your own (look online for recipes and starter kits).

Fermented Vegetables

Fermented Vegetables bring healthy microbes to the table! Many companies create raw and nourishing fermented foods like raw pickles and sauerkraut. Check the ingredients. Those found in jars and sold in stores will not give you healthy benefits. Unless it says raw and fermented, they are often made with vinegar, table salt, and are highly pasteurized. Pasteurization kills ALL bacteria and enhances shelf life. Fermented vegetables (and pickles) are extremely easy to make. There is a wealth of information online about fermented vegetables and how to make them.

Kimchi

Kimchi is a Korean version of sauerkraut. It's very spicy and sour. Not only does it have great gut-building bacteria, it's also full of calcium and Vitamins A, C and B1. This is a great probiotic food to include as a staple in your meals. Experiment with the different levels of spiciness. If someone doesn't have an appetite, give them a little bit of sauerkraut or Kimchi. This helps enhance taste buds to give them a desire for food again.

Yogurt

Yogurt is possibly one of the most widely known probiotic food. Be aware when selecting a yogurt. Find an organic, grass fed/grass finished plain (not sweetened) yogurt that has live-cultures for maximum health benefits. You can also easily make your own if you have access to raw milk. Frozen yogurt is devoid of beneficial bacteria. Pasteurized and sweetened yogurts are void of benefits as well.

Miso Paste

Miso Paste is a great digestive aid and commonly used in macrobiotic cooking. It's easy to make a soup, dressing or sauce. For soup, add miso paste to warm water and then add your favorite vegetables. You can use it as a dressing base and to add that umami flavor to sauces. A little goes a long way!

Sauerkraut

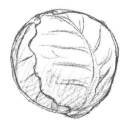

See next page for Sauerkraut benefits and recipe.
Not a complete list of fermented foods.

How to Make Sauerkraut
(Fermented Cabbage or Vegetables)

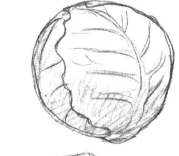

Ingredients:
* 1 head of Organic Cabbage (any variety, green or purple)
* 1 TBSP Celtic Sea Salt
* 1 half gallon or gallon glass wide-mouth jar

Directions:

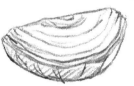

1. Use one fresh head of organic cabbage.

2. Peel off 3-5 leaves and save for later.

3. Finely chop the cabbage.

4. Place in bowl and add about 1/2 TBSP salt to chopped cabbage. ONLY USE Celtic Sea Salt or Himalayan Salt.

5. With clean hands, squish and massage cabbage. Massage until the cabbage feels soft or wilted.

6. Let the wilted cabbage sit for about 10 minutes.

7. Pack cabbage tightly into clean, sterilized (with just hot water and simple soap such as Bronners®) wide-mouth jar.

8. Cover with whole cabbage leaves and compress with a weight.

9. Cover with a cloth and secure with a rubber band.

10. Place in a cool and dark area (put the date on the outside).

11. After four days, peel off cabbage leaves and taste.

12. You can either place the leaves back on top and cover with cloth to continue fermenting, OR place in a glass jar with a tight lid and refrigerate.

Always use clean tongs or utensils to remove sauerkraut. The salt causes water to leach out of the leaves, and then naturally occurring bacteria on the leaves cause a fermentation that turns the cabbage into sauerkraut and preserves it. The salt also acts as a preservative.

Start by eating 1 tsp of your homemade Sauerkraut 2-3 times per day and notice your digestion. Then slowly increase to 1-2 tsp per meal every day. Eventually you will CRAVE Sauerkraut!

The beneficial bacteria of fermented foods (such as sauerkraut) helps with the digestive/gastrointestinal health of your body. By eating a little sauerkraut with each meal, the enzymes in the sauerkraut increase nutrition absorption and ease digestion. Sauerkraut contains Vitamin C, Vitamin K, iron, and is a great source of fiber. The fermentation process increases the vitamins, minerals, and health benefits of cabbage.

During the first week of the fermentation process, there is the most growth in beneficial bacteria. If you choose, you can add more probiotics to your sauerkraut. Mix 1/4 tsp of your favorite probiotic powder and add to sauerkraut for more probiotic power. You can also add sauerkraut juice from previous batches into your new batch. Make sure the brine is all the way to the top.

If you do not have enough brine, you can create a brine:
Add 1-1/2 TBSP Celtic Sea Salt or Himalayan Salt to
1 quart (32 oz) Purified Water

Or use the ratio: 1 tsp brine to 16 oz of PURIFIED (not tap) water.

The Benefits of Sauerkraut Keep Going!

Pirate Approved! Story has it that Captain C. Cook brought barrels of sauerkraut aboard his ship to prevent his men from getting scurvy! Scurvy is a vitamin C deficiency which killed many sailors during long voyages.

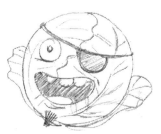

* Reduces bloating, flatulence and pain in irritable bowel syndrome.

* Contains antioxidants such as glutathione which can help fight off free radicals.

* Increases the beneficial flora in the intestinal tract. Eat sauerkraut, especially if you take any antibiotics (re-builds the good flora that antibiotics kill).

* Sauerkraut has anti-inflammatory properties (works great for arthritis and joint pain).

* Can help you get over illness, colds, and flu quicker.

Start simple, experiment and embrace the fermented vegetables!

WARNING:
Adding too many probiotic foods at once can loosen your bowel movements. If you find that your bowel movements become too loose when incorporating probiotic foods, ease off just a little until they are solid again.

Start with 1-2 tsp a DAY (if you are not used to probiotic foods). Then slowly build up to 1-2 TBSP per meal. If you find that you have issues with constipation, increasing the amount of probiotic foods (along with ample purified water and organic fibrous foods) may help bring natural constipation relief. Always go slowly with new foods to see how they assimilate in your body. Remember, everyone is different and what works for others may not work for you.

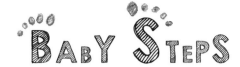

 List the probiotic foods that appeal to you, and commit to eating or trying one this week:

 Find the probiotic/fermented food that appeals to you most and incorporate one of them in small amounts on a daily basis. Feel free to mix it up. The wider the variety of your probiotic foods, the larger the variety of beneficial bacterial you will introduce to your gut:

 If you do well with the probiotic foods and enjoy them, begin to incorporate small amounts into 2-3 meals or snacks a day:

Understand Your Food, Understand Your Mood

Food/Mood Journal

At this point, you now have a good idea of how the Upgrade process works. You understand blood sugar stabilizing food combinations (Magic Trio Combinations), and the importance of Upgrading your foods and beverages. So what's your next step? In order to be successful, it helps to understand HOW your food affects you. As you track the foods you eat and the moods you feel, you will begin to understand your patterns.

I can't tell you how many clients resist the Food/Mood Journal. This is a common finding in my live programs. So many participants tell me "I eat REALLY healthy" and still don't understand why they have certain health issues. Once they start reading ingredients, the light switch is turned on. Once they write in their Food/Mood Journal, the ah-ha's start coming...the lights are so bright, they have to wear shades!

With everything in this process, start with baby steps. First, jot down what you eat. If that feels simple enough, start to fill out another category in the Food/Mood Journal. Use template on the next page or create a system that works for you. Some people use their phone, others a spreadsheet, and others like to write it down by hand. Use any format that suits you. Stick with it...this is your magic mirror of digestive awareness.

Simple Food/Mood Journal

1. Day Time	2. Mouth Hunger or Belly Hunger	3. Type and Quantity	4. Is the food you ate different from what you craved?	5. What were you doing while eating?	6. How do you feel after eating?
Example: Mon 4pm	Mouth Hunger	1 large bag of Chips, Chocolate Milk & Granola	Wanted a burger	Driving Home	Very tired & bloated
Tues Noon	Belly Hunger	Large Salad from Cafeteria	Pizza	At Desk	Good

1. Write down the day and time.
2. Notice if it's 'Mouth Hunger' (Bored/Emotional eating) or 'Belly Hunger' (grumble in the tummy)
3. Type and quantity of food (just an approximate) a bag of..., bowl of... package of... plate of...
4. Is the food you ate different from what you craved?
5. If so, what did you crave? Write it down <——— Importance of cravings (see Craveology page 35)
6. What were you doing while eating? Sitting at a table, watching TV, driving, working, etc.?
7. How do you feel after eating? Tired, craving more, satisfied, bloated, acidic, etc.?

5 - Blood-Sugarology

Willing to investigate a littler further? If so, fill out this Food/Mood Journal for one week.

1. Date/Time	Mon 4pm
2. Mouth or Belly Hunger	Mouth Hunger
3. Type/Quantity	1 Large bag of chips 16 oz Chocolate Milk 1 Granola Bar
4. Is this What you Craved?	Kinda
5. If not... What did you Crave?	Would have been nice to sit down for a meal. A big burger or pizza sounded nice. Too much effort, just grabbed some snacks.
6. Where is your food from? Ingredients	Grocery Store. Ingredients: Ugh - read them after I ate items, obviously need to look before, Bad Oil's and Refined Sugars, and ingredients I don't understand
7. What were you doing?	Driving Home
8. Did you Chew?	Probably Not
9. How do you feel after?	Very Tired and Bloated
10. How do you feel 1.5 - 2 Hours after? *set timer	Wanting something else to snack on, mouth hunger, but stomach doesn't feel too good.

Use a Journal or digital format to keep track of these questions for a week. Create it in a format that works for you! You can download the food/mood journal from www.upgradeology.com

1. Day/Time
2. Is it 'Mouth Hunger' (Bored/Emotional eating) or 'Belly Hunger' (grumble in the tummy)
3. Type and quantity of food (just an approximate) a bag of, bowl of... package of... plate of...
4. Is the food you ate different from what you craved?
5. If so, what did you crave? Write it down <——— Importance of cravings (see Craveology, page 35)
6. Where is your food from? (Homemade, boxed, canned, restaurant, fast food? If homemade, where are the ingredients from? Mono (single) ingredients, part of a box (i.e. a boxed cake where you add egg and water).
7. What were you doing while eating? Sitting at a table, watching TV, driving, working, etc.?
8. Do you chew your food a few times before gulping it down, or do you take the time to really chew your food?
9. How do you feel after eating -- tired, craving more, satisfied, bloated, acidic, etc.?
10. How do you feel 1.5 – 2 hours later (set timer)? Sluggish, energized, hungry, headache, etc.?

In Chapter 5 we discussed:

* The Magic Trio Combinations and how they stabilize your blood sugar
* The importance of the Sauce
* How to create your own Upgraded versions
  of your favorite sauces and spreads
* Releasing the diet mentality
* Multiple hidden names of MSG
* The importance of eating quality foods
* Nourishing Fats
* How Breakfast and Snacks will balance your
  blood sugar and keep you motivated to continue to Upgrade
* The difference between Fast Carbs, Fruit Carbs and Slow Carbs
* An easy way to keep Upgrading by having your "Gotta Go Bag"
* The healing benefits of Enzymes and Probiotic Foods
* Understand your food and understanding your mood

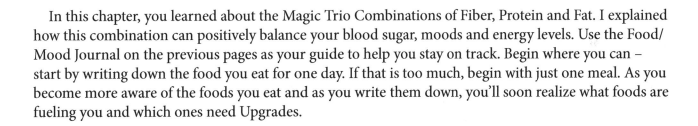

In this chapter, you learned about the Magic Trio Combinations of Fiber, Protein and Fat. I explained how this combination can positively balance your blood sugar, moods and energy levels. Use the Food/Mood Journal on the previous pages as your guide to help you stay on track. Begin where you can – start by writing down the food you eat for one day. If that is too much, begin with just one meal. As you become more aware of the foods you eat and as you write them down, you'll soon realize what foods are fueling you and which ones need Upgrades.

Chapter 6 will guide you through the Upgrade process. Whether you want to find delicious options for your favorite (yet damaging) comfort foods, decrease your daily caffeine intake, or just find out what Upgraded foods are all about, this next chapter will show you how to successfully Upgrade your food and beverages. You will find that you have a wide variety of satisfying and nourishing options to choose from. Remember to take one baby step at a time. Experiment and play around with what works best for your personal taste and lifestyle.

"Man often becomes what he believes himself to be.
If I keep on saying to myself that I cannot do a certain thing,
it is possible that I may end by really becoming incapable of doing it.
On the contrary, if I shall have the belief that I can do it,
I shall surely acquire the capacity to do it,
even if I may not have it at the beginning."
- Mahatma Gandhi

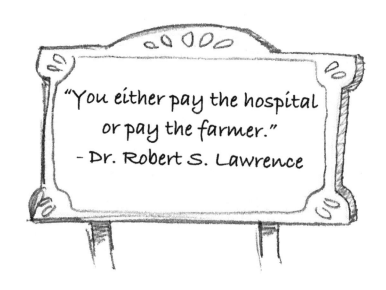

"You either pay the hospital or pay the farmer."
- Dr. Robert S. Lawrence

6 Upgradeolgy

How to Satisfy Your Cravings With The Upgrade Process

Upgrades

An Upgrade replaces a food that is toxic, fake or harmful for a natural, healthier and more nutritious version without deprivation. When you see tempting, delicious food that is filled with chemicals and gunk, ask yourself the following question: how can I Upgrade this food and make it with REAL, nourishing ingredients? This takes away the feeling that you are missing out on your favorite food. Become creative in the kitchen or with your shopping intentions. The Upgrade process teaches you how to create a delicious and satisfying version of whatever foods call your name.

This chapter is the belly of it all. Upgrades keep your belly and mind happy and satisfied. Upgrades can be done many different ways. Have an 'I Can list' (page 182) with you at all times so you stay committed to your Upgrades. As discussed in the previous chapter, upgrading to nourishing food saves you money and is a long-term investment in your health and well-being. See Shopping Guide on page 187 for more money-saving tips.

Easy Upgrades to get you started

Old	UPGRADED
White Rice	Organic Brown Rice
Refined Sugar	Organic Coconut Sugar
Artificial Sweeteners	Organic Green Stevia Powder
Vegetable/Soy/Canola Oil	Organic Extra Virgin Coconut Oil
Hydrogenated Oil	Organic Extra Virgin Coconut Oil
Table Salt	Celtic Sea Salt

Use the Upgrades Chart and Conversions in this Chapter. When you Upgrade fast food/processed frankenfoods to REAL food or a nourishing homemade version, you take positive steps in the healing direction. You don't have to Upgrade these foods all at once. **Take ONE baby step at a time!** Remember to pick and choose Upgrades that fit your personal lifestyle and needs...

Upgrades Options:

1st Option - Upgrade to higher quality food wherever possible.

For example: if your dinner or lunch routine is to hit the fast food drive-thru, find a higher quality restaurant that serves healthier, nourishing menu items. It's important to start asking about the ingredients in the food. Do they use any kind of sugar, corn syrup, MSG or artificial sweeteners? What kind of oil do they cook in?

Remember that fat-free, low-fat, diet anything, reduced calorie, etc. are NOT healthier options. When the fat is taken out of the food (**fat = flavor**) artificial ingredients replace them. It's HEALTHIER to have real butter than it is to have margarine. It's HEALTHIER to have sprouted whole grain bread than the gluten-free options with binders and sugars available en masse. **REAL food is always more nourishing than FAKE food!**

Old	UPGRADED
Fast Food	Quality restaurant with organic ingredients
Cheap Pizza	Quality restaurant or homemade
Margarine	Real Butter
Low-Fat Yogurt	Plain Grass Fed Yogurt
Artificial Sweetener	Upgraded Sweeteners (Organic Stevia)
Canola Oil/Vegetable Oil	Coconut Oil, Butter or Ghee

2nd Option - Organic or organic frozen

For example: if you bring frozen "diet" meals to work for lunch, shop around and Upgrade to a high quality organic frozen meal instead. Shop at markets that carry these items – this eases the temptation to buy the old version.

Old	UPGRADED
Low-Fat Frozen Entrées	Organic Frozen Entrées
Take Out/Fast Food	Organic Frozen Entrées
General Frozen Foods	Organics or natural/simple ingredients

The best way to know what truly quality food is - thoroughly read the package and INGREDIENTS. The ingredients will eventually help guide your decision.

3rd Option - Homemade with simple ingredients

You can find ANY recipe online. Even using generic ingredients will often be an Upgrade from what any fast food and most chain restaurants serve. If you like to cook, this is an excellent way to start Upgrading. There are so many options in many of the natural grocery stores where you don't have to make everything from scratch, but you can still see what ingredients go into your food.

Old	UPGRADED
Fast Food/Take Out	Homemade with simple ingredients
Greasy Restaurants Comfort Food	Homemade comfort food

4th Option to aspire to - Homemade with organic ingredients

Love to cook? Interested in cooking more? This is the section for you. Take your favorite recipes and begin to convert the ingredients to organic and quality ingredients. You will find your food tastes amazing and your body will digest it with greater ease. There are so many foods that I love to eat that make me ill when eating out, and I do just fine when I make them myself.

Old	UPGRADED
Restaurants	Homemade with clean quality ingredients
Pre-packaged or frozen	Homemade with clean quality ingredients

Cooking can take a lot of time so consciously make a lot of leftovers. Freeze them yourself for those grab and go days. You can cook a week's worth of food, package it up yourself, and have better quality food for an entire week. See Cooking Strategies in Chapter 8 for more tips!

❊ Remember the Fiber, Protein, and Fat Mantra (Magic Trio Combinations)!

Magic Trio Combinations (**see Chapter 5, page 101**) include fiber, protein, and fat. This combination helps stabilize your food cravings and blood sugar levels.

Breakfast Foods

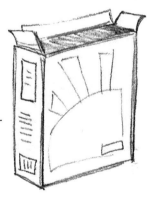

All boxed cereals are processed foods. However, the more natural ones will have much less refined sugars, flours, artificial additives, and toxic oils/chemicals included in them. All cereals go through a process that heats ingredients to an extremely high heat to make them a slurry; they are then flattened (flakes) or extruded (shapes) cooked over high heat again and coated with a variety of ingredients to create the crispy nature of it. This is not natural, but if you love cereal, it's helpful to look for cereals with the least amount of ingredients, and without refined sugar, artificial colors or flavorings.

Old	UPGRADED
Boxed Cereal	Organic cereals with minimal ingredients.
Bread/Toast/English Muffin	Find an organic sprouted brand with minimal ingredients that you understand.
French Toast/Pancakes/Waffles	There are a few frozen ones that have decent ingredients. These are best made homemade with ingredients you choose. Many Organic or Farm-to-table and sugar-conscious restaurants also make tasty options.
Instant or quick cooking hot cereals	Find the whole grains such as Organic gluten-free rolled oats, steel cut oats, organic brown rice, etc. Soak overnight and then heat up on the stovetop. You can also cook them overnight in a slow cooker.

A client calls this recipe her:

"Morning Apple Pie"

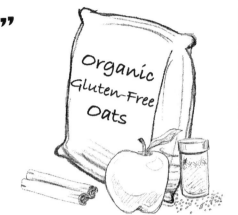

Ingredients
* 1 cup organic gluten-free rolled oats
* 1 small organic apple, peeled and chopped
* 1 tsp cinnamon
* 2 cups purified water
* Celtic Sea Salt to taste

Directions:
1. Place all ingredients into the slow cooker and give it a little stir.
2. Turn slow cooker to low and cook overnight.
3. In the morning, open up and prepare for yum.

Protein Shakes

READ ALL INGREDIENTS! Protein shakes of ALL kinds are notorious for having hidden GMOs, soy, sugar, and artificial flavors and sweeteners. Even some of the Organic brands are filled with hidden sugars and artificial flavors.

If you drink protein shakes, then you probably love the convenience of them. That's ok - find ones with the cleanest ingredients. Go to the health food store and ask an attendant to help you.

NOTE: Without the artificial ingredients or sugar in protein powders, they will taste chalky and extremely bland or earthy. Do your research, get simple ingredients, and create your own protein shake. I'm shocked at some of the holistic folks who have put out their own protein powders on the market. Even their ingredients are iffy sometimes. Become a committed label reader. Think about what people had for breakfast 100 years ago. We didn't have all these shakes and bars and uber-convenient foods. You CAN still have them – just recognize what kind of convenience you are going after.

What to look for in a Protein Powder:
* Certified Organic
* Non-GMO
* No Refined Sugar or Artificial Sweetener/Coloring/Flavoring

*Add your own Upgraded Sweetener or fresh fruit. **See Upgraded Sweeteners on pages 77, 83-85.**

Dairy

Old	UPGRADED
Low-Fat/Fat-Free Flavored Yogurt:	Organic Grass Fed Plain Yogurt or Greek Yogurt - add your own fruit and/or natural sweetener.
Low-Fat/Fat-Free Milk:	Organic Grass Fed Whole Milk. Dilute it yourself with water and add your own natural sweetener.
Whey:	Organic Grass Fed (without other ingredients or sugar)
Cream/Sour Cream/Cottage Cheese/Cream Cheese, etc.:	Upgrade to Certified Organic and Grass Fed.
Any Dairy Product:	With dairy, it's essential to purchase certified organic and grass fed items to avoid ingesting harmful hormones and antibiotics (which create inflammation and dis-harmony in the body).
Cheese:	Organic Grass Fed Cheese (raw is excellent). Goat and Sheep Cheese are also excellent options.
Non-Dairy Substitutes: Non-Dairy Creamers:	Read the ingredients - these are all fake ingredients! Try coconut or nut butters instead. Many people who cannot tolerate dairy do well with Goat or Sheep dairy.
Nut/Seed/Coconut Milks:	Best homemade or find organic unsweetened milk minimally processed with few ingredients – add your own natural sweetener.
Soy Milk:	Upgrade to an organic nut/seed/coconut milk. Soy milk is not the health food we once thought it was. (See soy on page 89)
Vegan Cheese:	Nutritional Yeast or a Fermented Seed Cheese (See Recipe section). Many of the almond/soy/vegan cheeses are FULL of toxic ingredients.
Ice Cream:	You can find recipes and easily make ice cream at home. I love to freeze bananas, and then blend them with blueberries and nut butter to create my own ice cream. Most of the time you won't even need added sweeteners when bananas are your base. Experiment for yourself. See Banana Ice Cream recipe on page 259.

Meals

Old	UPGRADED
Burger:	Grass Fed and an Organic Bun. Farm-to-table restaurants or homemade with quality ingredients.
Canned Chili/Soups:	Organic version or make your own.
Comfort Food:	Farm-to-table restaurants or restaurants with clean, quality ingredients. Home made.
Fast Foods:	Upgrade to a quality restaurant. Upgrade to organic frozen foods. Make a large quantity of homemade food, portion out your meals, and freeze.
Fried Foods (French Fries/ Fried Chicken, etc.)	If you have to have fried food, make it yourself with coconut oil or pasture raised animal fat. These are the only fats that can tolerate high heat. All the oils used to fry foods in 99% of restaurants are toxic oils. You can also bake items until crispy for a similar texture.
Frozen Dinners:	Upgrade to organics. Make a large quantity of homemade food, portion out your meals, and freeze.
Mashed Potatoes:	Use organic potatoes, sweet potatoes, cauliflower, celery root or millet as a substitute. Cook, add butter, garlic, sea salt, and yum! (Recipe on page 242)
Microwave Meals:	Upgrade to stove top, toaster oven, or oven-cooked. If the microwave is your ONLY option for heating up meals: make sure meals are in paper, ceramic or glass (never plastic – plastic will leach toxins into your food). Then thaw out the food as best you can in the refrigerator or counter-top and cook for the minimal amount of time possible to warm food. See Chapter 8 for more Cooking tips!
Restaurants: Italian, Mexican, American, Indian, Asian, etc.:	Ask them about their ingredients and see for yourself if they use quality ingredients. Ask them what oils they use, do they cook with MSG, artificial ingredients, sweeteners, sugar, corn syrup, etc.
Pasta:	Organic brown rice or quinoa pasta, spaghetti squash, kelp noodles, zucchini cut like little spirals. Get creative with pasta.
Pizza:	Organic, quality restaurant or homemade version. MOST pizza/pasta sauce has sugar in it.
Rice:	Organic brown rice, basmati rice
Bread:	Organic sprouted or sourdough. Minimal ingredients or homemade.

Snacks

Old	UPGRADED
Chips:	Upgrade to organics, and find the ones made with coconut oil (it's the only oil that is safe at high heat). Bake your own using root vegetables, coconut oil, sea salt, and your favorite seasoning.
Chocolate:	Find chocolates made with coconut sugar (there are quite a few on the market these days and they are DEE-LICIOUS). Remember that Agave is fructose and contributes to diabetes and obesity. You can also make your own chocolate with Cacao powder, cacao butter, and your sweetener of choice. See Chocolate Chip Cookies recipe on page 151 and Hot Chocolate recipe on page 30.
Dried Fruit:	Get Organic, read ingredients, and make sure there are no additives, sulfur, etc. Note: Cranberries will almost always have sugar in them.
Flavored Yogurt:	Get PLAIN, Organic Grass Fed and Grass Finished. Add your own toppings and Upgraded Sweeteners.
Granola:	Find an organic version. Some are now made with coconut sugar which are excellent. I also enjoy making my own. It's easy to do - See Granola Bars in recipe section on page 256.
Popcorn:	Make your own. Microwave popcorn is full of toxic ingredients. Movie popcorn isn't any better (ask to see what oil they use and what their 'butter flavoring' is made from if you are not convinced). Make your own (page 90) with coconut oil, butter, or animal fat. Be sure to always purchase NON-GMO popping corn..
Protein Bars:	There are a few out there with clean organic ingredients. Do your research.
Snack Foods/Cookies/ Candy Bars/Chips, etc.:	Upgrade to an organic version. More and more are showing up on the shelves because people are demanding them. Some of the RAW food snacks have extremely high quality ingredients. Some of them are replacing agave for coconut sugar. Keep your eye out and make shopping at the health food store an adventure!
Cakes, Cookies, Pastries, Pies, Doughnuts, etc.	Find the best quality version you can. Some of the RAW foods are an excellent Upgrade and taste delicious. For the most part, many of my clients will make what they desire from scratch. They feel confident in their Upgrades and they taste delicious. Do the best you can with the sweet stuff. Experiment with baking (see Recipe Alterations beginning on page 150) and see what amazing delicacies you can create.

Condiments, Condiments, Condiments

Most common brand condiments and dressings are FULL of refined sugars and other gunk. Sugar will be listed in numerous ways: GMO Gluten, MSG, Artificial Ingredients, Soy, Corn Syrup, etc.

#1: Find an organic version - even this Upgrade can be enough for many people.

#2: Look up the ingredients and using the Conversion chart (page 152), create an Upgraded version yourself.

Soy Sauce: Use Coconut Aminos or find an Organic, NON-GMO version. Most soy sauces are quickly cooked and full of MSG and other undesirables – read the bottle and ingredients to find out how your favorite soy sauce is processed. There are organic versions that are made with quality ingredients found in the health food store.

Create a condiment tray for your table so that you and your family can personalize every meal. A turn table or 'Lazy Susan' is perfect for storing all the different condiments on your table. See How to Upgrade Your Family on page 157.

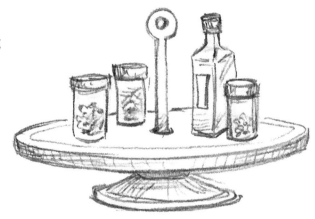

Here are some condiments worthy of experimenting with. Feel free to add your favorites to this list. Use organic whenever possible. Look for those with minimal ingredients, no additives/preservatives or ingredients you don't understand.

Spices
Basil
Garlic
Cumin
Ginger
Thyme
Oregano
Turmeric
Cinnamon
Curry Powder
Garam Masala Spice Mix

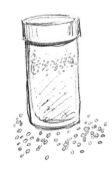

Heat
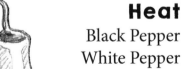
Black Pepper
White Pepper
Chili Powder
Chili Flakes
Cayenne
Paprika

Salts
Celtic Sea Salt
Himalayan Salt

Nuts and Seeds

Nut Butters: Tahini, Cashew, Almond, etc.
Nuts: Pine, Brazil, Cashews, Walnuts, Almonds, Pistachios, etc.
Seeds: Pumpkin, Sunflower, Sesame, Flax, Chia, Hemp

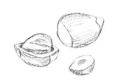

Nurturing Oil & Fats

Extra Virgin Coconut Oil or Butter
Extra Virgin Olive Oil
Grass Fed Butter
Avocado

Sweeteners

Raw Honey
Coconut Sugar
Coconut Nectar
Brown Rice Syrup
Grade B Maple Syrup
Homemade Apple Sauce
Green Stevia Leaf or Stevia Liquid
Fruit: Apples, Dates, Figs, Raisins, etc.

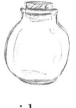

Sea Vegetables

Dulse flakes
Nori sheets
Kelp flakes
Wakame
Kombu
Hijiki

Sauces

Pesto
Hot Sauces
Olive Paste
Salad Dressings
Tomato sauce
Coconut Amino Acids

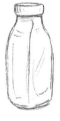

Other

Spirulina
Coconut Milk
Nutritional Yeast
Raw Sauerkraut
Grated Daikon Radish
Pasture Raised Eggs (yolk)
Sprouts: Sunflower, Mung, etc.
Plain Grass Fed Greek or Regular Yogurt

Zing

Mustard
Miso Paste
Uemboshi Plum
RAW Apple Cider Vinegar

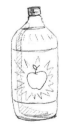

* Not a complete list. More 'make-it-yourself ideas on the next page and page 108.

* Explore, Create & Use Organic Whenever Possible!

Make Your Own Dressing

1. Mix 1-3 parts unrefined organic oil to 1 part organic vinegar or organic citrus juice.

2. Add organic seasonings and choice of organic herbs or spices until the flavors blend well.

3. Shake and let stand 10 minutes before serving.

Unrefined Oils:

Cold-Pressed Sesame oil

Cold-Pressed Flax Oil

Extra Virgin Coconut Oil

Extra Virgin Olive Oil

* Note: The above oils must be **unrefined** in order to avoid unhealthy results. In addition, flax and all polyunsaturated oils should be '**fresh**', recently cold-pressed, kept cool, and in a dark colored bottle to protect from light and oxidation.

Zing:

Umeboshi plum

Miso paste

Lemon

Lime

Bell Peppers

Grated Ginger

Coconut Aminos

RAW Apple Cider Vinegar

Juice:

(FRESH Squeezed):

Lemon

Lime

Grapefruit

Orange

Sweet:

Raw Honey

Maple Syrup

Stevia

Fruit

Coconut Sugar

Coconut Nectar

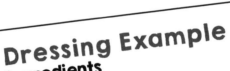

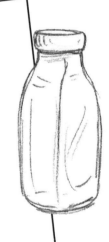

Dressing Example
Ingredients
* ½ cup Olive Oil
* ½ cup RAW Apple Cider Vinegar
* ½ Fresh squeezed lemon
* 1 medium avocado
* 2 TBSP Coconut Sugar
* 2 TBSP fresh chopped basil
* 2 TBSP freshly grated ginger
* 1 tsp Celtic Sea Salt (or to taste)

Directions:
1. Place all ingredients in blender (use ½ tsp of Celtic Sea Salt to begin).
2. Blend until smooth.
3. Add more Celtic Sea Salt to taste.
4. Store in a glass container in the refrigerator.

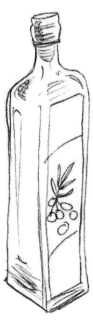

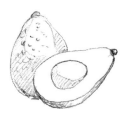
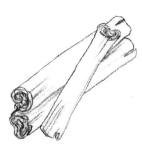
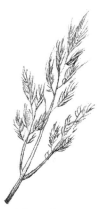

Creamy:

Avocado

Nut/Seed Butters

Whole Grains

Yogurt

Coconut Butter

Coconut Oil

Cooked Organic Veggies

Salt:

Celtic Sea Salt

Himalayan Salt

Seaweed

Spice:

Anise

Curry

Cayenne

Cinnamon

Coriander

Clove

Nutmeg

Cumin

Cardamom, etc.

Herbs:

Basil

Thyme

Rosemary

Tarragon

Marjoram

Oregano

Dill

Sage

Mint

Ginger

Chives

Onion

Garlic, etc.

Make Your Own Dressing

Ingredients

* Oil:_____

* Zing:_____

* Juice:_____

* Sweet:_____

* Creamy:_____

* Salts:_____

* Spices:_____

* Herbs:_____

* Other:_____

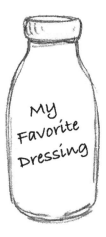

Directions:

1. Place all ingredients in blender.
2. Blend until desired texture.
3. Taste and alter until desired taste.

* **Explore, Create & Use Organic Whenever Possible.**
* **See Recipe Section for more Upgrade options!**

Beverages

Old	UPGRADED
Frappa Rhappa Momos (you know, frozen coffee drinks) or Lattes, Americanos, etc.:	Organic Fair Trade Coffee, Chicory Root or Organic Teas
Coffee drinks:	Organic Fair Trade Coffee, Chicory Root, Organic Teas
Soda:	Bubbly Water, Mineral Water, plus sweetener and or fruit, Kombucha
Bubbly Water/Mineral Water/Natural Club Soda:	Get a bottle of Mineral water, and add a squeeze of lemon or lime and mint leaves. This is a refreshing, non-alcoholic drink to sip at parties while others drink cocktails.
Fruit Juice:	Make your own or buy FRESH from a Juice Bar
Energy Drinks:	Green Tea, Kombucha, Coconut Water, Lemon/Lime Water, diluted Organic Apple Cider Vinegar. After a while you won't need those 'energy drinks' if you get enough sleep and start using real ingredients.
Mocha, Chocolate Milk:	Find chocolate made with coconut sugar. Make your own using raw cacao, cacao butter, and/or coconut oil, and your favorite Upgraded Sweetener.
Vitamin Water:	Save your money! Get away from artificial sweeteners and make your own vitamin water. Start with purified water and add your favorite fruits to the water. The water absorbs the fruits' flavors, nutrients, and minerals. Add a variety of berries or squeeze a little lemon or lime into your water. The fruit makes the water look beautiful and taste delicious. You will end up craving this healthy vitamin water far more instead of the fake stuff.

Sweetened Iced Tea Options:

* Find an organic tea that you enjoy. Simmer water, add tea bag, and steep. Once the tea cools, place it in the refrigerator to chill (*or add purified water ice cubes to cool it down and dilute).

* For sun tea, find a large clear glass container and fill with purified water. Use 1 teabag for every 1-2 cups of water. Place the glass container in a sunny window or with a lid outside for 2-4 hours. When it looks like the color of tea, it's ready. Bring sun tea inside and place in refrigerator to chill.

* You can also add teabags to water and set it in the refrigerator overnight to steep. For 6 cups of water, add 2 tea bags. After you make iced tea the first time, you'll realize if you like your tea stronger or weaker. If you want the tea weaker, simply add more purified water. If you want it stronger, use more tea bags.

Sweeten your Iced or Sun tea:	Add your favorite Upgraded Sweetener (See pages 77, 83-85 for ideas). You can also add fresh herbs such as mint. Add the herbs with the tea bags or after you make the tea.
Ice:	*If you don't have a way of making ice from purified water, then stick your tea in the refrigerator until it's cold. Most ice (unless filtered) is tap water. See Water Section (page 46) for more information about tap water.
Electrolytes Juice/Sports Drink:	Organic Coconut water and/or electrolyte enhanced water. For additional flavoring, add fruit or your favorite natural sweetener (always check ingredients).

How to Upgrade Your Favorite Drink

The chart listed below is a great way to Upgrade your favorite beverage slowly. If you care for a child, an elder, or secretly Upgrade drinks that you serve to family and friends, this process is a great way to do it without the shock of going cold turkey. You can use this method with food, too!

For example, if you are a soda drinker:
Day 1: drink **90% of the soda** you would normally consume and then begin to ADD **10% sparkling mineral water.**
The chart below will help you slowly transition to an Upgraded drink.

WARNING: When you immediately cut out an addictive drink that you consume on a regular basis, the process can end up backfiring. Trust me on this one. It takes a little bit of planning but it really works. Begin to slowly dilute the drink you've loved for so long, and slowly transition to an Upgraded beverage. **It's a win-win strategy!** Give it a try!

Beverage UPGRADE Chart

Day 1:	90% old	10% NEW Upgrade
Day 2:	80% old	20% NEW Upgrade
Day 3:	70% old	30% NEW Upgrade
Day 4:	60% old	40% NEW Upgrade
Day 5:	50% old	50% NEW Upgrade
Day 6:	40% old	60% NEW Upgrade
Day 7:	30% old	70% NEW Upgrade
Day 8:	20% old	80% NEW Upgrade
Day 9:	10% old	90% NEW Upgrade
Day 10:		100% NEW Upgrade

If caffeine is kicking your butt, kick your caffeine and coffee habit **gradually** with these helpful tips coming up next.

Quirky or Perky?

How Caffeine Affects Your Body. Most of us have been there. The afternoon hits and your energy drags so you turn to coffee (or soda or an energy drink) to get through the rest of your day. Over time, that little pick-me-up becomes two or three, and soon you are completely reliant upon caffeinated beverages. But what does caffeine actually do to your body?

First, caffeine increases your stress hormones! Those "jittery" feelings when you've had too much caffeine are physical symptoms of anxiety. Stress hormones have also been linked to stomach issues, insomnia, and can even affect your immune system. By increasing your stress hormones, you actually decrease your ability to handle daily stress.

While most of us equate caffeine with anxiety or irritability, it can also be linked to depression. Think about it! Caffeine stimulates your body in ways that are unnatural. As your body comes down from that caffeine high, you can actually put yourself into a state of depression.

Caffeine increases your body's energy by creating a temporary boost in blood sugar, which leads to the production of too much insulin. This feeling is what creates the "crash" that's generally felt after drinking caffeinated beverages. This makes caffeine especially risky for people with diabetes or hypoglycemia, and can also lead to weight gain.

Caffeine also decreases your body's ability to absorb much-needed nutrients. Caffeine encourages your body to excrete essential nutrients like calcium, magnesium, and potassium through your urine. As you drink caffeine, your adrenal glands become exhausted and increase your risk for a variety of health problems.

Caffeine: Anything with the word caffeine in it - Cacao, Guarana Green/Black/White tea.

Function: To boost energy quickly

Found in: Sodas, 'energy drinks', diet and pain pills, and gum. It's also naturally found in chocolate, coffee, and some teas.

Side Effects: Many forms of caffeine can leach calcium from your bones. This does not mean that taking a calcium supplement will make up for this calcium loss. Lack of calcium can lead to infertility and osteoporosis. The natural forms of caffeine are much healthier for you (with fewer side effects).

Safer alternatives: Read ALL Ingredients on food and drink labels. If you need your morning coffee, Upgrade to an organic brand. If you drink decaf, opt for the 'Swiss water process'. Drink more water and switch to a calmer, soothing beverage such as **green tea** (contains beneficial antioxidants). We need our rituals. Coffee/caffeine is usually a morning ritual for many people. I honor that ritual for myself, and encourage my clients to also indulge in their warm, yummy morning drink ritual.

How to kick the caffeine habit without the headache!

Caffeine is a drug. If you don't believe that caffeine is a drug, then go cold turkey without caffeine for one day, and let me know how that goes for you. I don't recommend it, because you are bound to have a very difficult day with a splitting headache.

If you want to kick your caffeine habit, I highly recommend going off caffeine gradually. I created this chart (see below) because of my personal experiences with caffeine. I followed this chart every time I started drinking coffee again and needed to release my coffee habit. This process allowed me to slowly decrease my caffeine intake without miserable headaches and fatigue. Give it a try!

Take 7-10 days for this process. Start on a non-work day or your least demanding day. If you work Monday through Friday, then start on Saturday. As a result, you will be caffeine-free without putting your life on hold or suffering needless detox symptoms.

10 Day No-Withdrawal from Coffee Example

1. Upgrade your coffee to an Organic brand (fair trade if possible).

2. Get Organic Swiss Water Decaf, Herbal Tea or Chicory Root (as your decaf).

3. Upgrade anything you include in your coffee:
   * Upgrade regular or diet creamer to Organic Cream, Half and Half, Coconut Oil or Nut or Seed Milk. See dairy Upgrades on page 135.
   * Upgrade refined sugar to one of the Upgraded Sweeteners (pages 77, 83-85)
   * Add real flavorings such as Organic Vanilla Extract, Almond Extract, Mint Extract, etc.

4. If you purchase your coffee every day, try this helpful tip: measure out your cup by inches. Pour ½ less inch of regular coffee each day and replace it with ½ inch of decaf. Be very friendly with your barista and tip well. Let the barista know what you are doing and how much you appreciate their help.

5. Another option: get one cup of regular and one cup of decaf. Make your drink (according to the chart below) and then gift the other coffee to someone else.

Day 1:	90% regular	10% decaf, tea or chicory root
Day 2:	80% regular	20% decaf, tea or chicory root
Day 3:	70% regular	30% decaf, tea or chicory root
Day 4:	60% regular	40% decaf, tea or chicory root
Day 5:	50% regular	50% decaf, tea or chicory root
Day 6:	40% regular	60% decaf, tea or chicory root
Day 7:	30% regular	70% decaf, tea or chicory root
Day 8:	20% regular	80% decaf, tea or chicory root
Day 9:	10% regular	90% decaf, tea or chicory root
Day 10:		100% decaf, tea or chicory root

No With-drawl!

6 - Upgradeology

If you find you still need caffeine and enjoy tea, you can switch over to organic green tea. Caffeine does not effect everyone in the same way. I have some clients who are not willing to give up their monring cup of coffee. They love it and tell me that they don't feel any negative effects from it. In that case, they just Upgrade all of the ingredients (Orgnaic coffee beans, organic dairy or coconut oil and an Upgraded Sweetener) and I recommend that they have only one or two cups and consume it before 11am.

Caffeine Questions:

* How much caffeine do you consume and in what form?

* What is a caffeine Upgrade that would work for you?

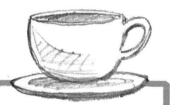

How to Upgrade

Gather all of the ingredients you will need.
In this case a client decided to turn in her expensive and chemical filled 20 oz morning mocha for a delicious homemade version.
* Organic Fair Trade Coffee
* Organic Decaf (Swiss water process decaf)
* Organic Extra Virgin Coconut Oil (or Organic Grass Fed milk/cream)
* Organic Coconut Sugar
* Organic Cacao Powder

Schedule your start date.
If you work Monday through Friday, begin your Beverage Upgrade on a Saturday. If you begin on a Monday and find that even 10% is too much to begin with, then the entire process can backfire. I've tried to reduce and restrict too much caffeine on a Monday. However, mid-day I couldn't think and ran to the nearest coffee shop and ordered a double of what I normally drank because I couldn't keep my eyes open. Don't let this happen to you! Begin on a day with the least amount of demands.

Create a chart.
Once you have all of your supplies, **create a chart with YOUR specifics.** Set yourself up for success from the very beginning. Make your Upgraded Beverage as delicious as possible and your transition will be smooth, delicious, and satisfying - another positive baby step to upgrading your health!

Upgrade in 3 STEPS

 Gather all of the ingredients you will need:

* *
* *
* *
* *
* *
* *

 Schedule your start date:

I will begin on: _____

3 **Create a chart or use this one:**

Day 1: 90% old_____   10% **Upgrade**_____

Day 2: 80% old_____   20% **Upgrade**_____

Day 3: 70% old_____   30% **Upgrade**_____

Day 4: 60% old_____   40% **Upgrade**_____

Day 5: 50% old_____   50% **Upgrade**_____

Day 6: 40% old_____   60% **Upgrade**_____

Day 7: 30% old_____   70% **Upgrade**_____

Day 8: 20% old_____   80% **Upgrade**_____

Day 9: 10% old_____   90% **Upgrade**_____

Day 10:   **100% Upgraded!**_____

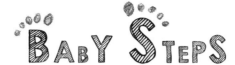

BABY STEPS

What is your favorite beverage? Write it here:

Do you think you would benefit from Upgrading it?

If you know you would benefit from an Upgraded beverage, what is the first ingredient you want to transition (i.e. refined sugar to organic coconut sugar)? Are you willing to plan and implement a 10 day transition (according to the chart on the previous page)? If not, be honest and list why you are not yet ready to Upgrade.

When are you willing to try one of the Beverage Upgrades?
Set a date, put it on your calendar and write down what you need to create a successful Upgrade.

Upgrade List

Now that you have a better idea of how you can Upgrade to more nourishing food and beverages, start thinking about the next step you want to take. Remember to add in Upgrades gradually. The Upgrade List next will keep you on track and set you up for success.

Week 1.
List your top 3 foods and/or drinks that you are willing to Upgrade:

1.

2.

3.

Now create **3 different Upgrades for each one**. Why 3 Upgrades? Because you'll need variety and **2 backups**, just in case the first one doesn't satisfy you.

Item #1
* Upgrade #1

* Upgrade #2

* Upgrade #3

Item #2
* Upgrade #1

* Upgrade #2

* Upgrade #3

Item #3
* Upgrade #1

* Upgrade #2

* Upgrade #3

Example: brand name chocolate bar

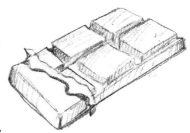

* **Upgrade #1:** Chocolate bar from the health food store made with organic cacao powder, cacao butter and coconut sugar.

* **Upgrade #2:** Homemade chocolate made with organic cacao powder, organic cacao powder, organic coconut sugar, and organic almonds.

* **Upgrade #3:** (Emergency back-up so you don't go back to the brand name chocolate bar) Organic dark chocolate with the least amount of sugar possible.

Keep this Upgrade List with you in an easy-to-find place. I write my list on my canvas shopping bag and use a fold up piece of paper for my wallet. When I pull out my money to pay at the market, I automatically see my list! If you have a plastic pocket in your wallet (i.e. for a driver's license or credit card) that you see all the time, keep your Upgrade List there. You may, or may not, be surprised when you **'forget'** to buy items on your list while at the market. You are probably too wrapped up in all the items that scream and beg to get into your cart and into your belly!

Here is an example of my list:

Old	UPGRADED
Bread	Homemade bean or quinoa bread (In emergency – organic sprouted or sourdough bread with organic, minimal and clean ingredients)
Chips	Kale chips, homemade chips, or chips made with coconut oil
Cookies	Homemade Almond Cookies or Almond Biscotti (see recipe section)
Crunchy	Carrots, jicama, bell peppers, apples, homemade popcorn, upgraded chips
Yogurt	Sheep or Goat Yogurt (or grass fed plain yogurt) or mashed Banana
Hearty	Organic nuts and seeds (dry roasted or raw/sprouted with sea salt)
Chocolate	Version made with coconut sugar or Homemade
Ice Cream	Blended frozen banana with frozen cherries, nuts, and seeds
Latte	Chicory root or green tea with coconut sugar and coconut oil
Mocha	Chicory root (or tea), cacao powder, coconut butter and coconut sugar

Recipe Alterations

At the beginning of this book, I promised you that you **don't** have to give up your favorite foods or cravings. Instead, just **Upgrade** them. **This section is for those who enjoy cooking.** Start by taking your favorite recipes and convert FAKE harmful ingredients into **REAL** nourishing, quality ingredients.

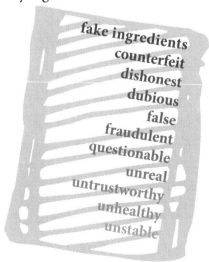

fake ingredients
counterfeit
dishonest
dubious
false
fraudulent
questionable
unreal
untrustworthy
unhealthy
unstable

Real Ingredients
* Authentic
* Legitimate
* Original
* True
* Bona Fide
* de Facto (in reality)
* In The Flesh
* Irrefutable
* LIVE
* Unaffected

UPGRADED Recipe Example:

Chocolate Chip Cookies

Original Recipe

* 2 1/4 cups all-purpose flour
* 1/2 tsp baking soda
* 1 cup butter

* 1/2 cup sugar
* 1 cup packed light-brown sugar
* 1 tsp salt
* 2 TBSP vanilla extract
* 2 eggs
* 2 cups (12 oz) chocolate chips

Upgraded Recipe (All Organic if possible)

* 2 1/2 cups Upgraded flour (see next page)
* 1/2 tsp aluminum-free baking soda
* 1 cup grass-fed unsalted butter or ghee
  Or extra Virgin Coconut Oil
* 1/2 cup Coconut Sugar
  plus 1 more cup of Coconut Sugar or Maple Syrup
* 1 tsp Celtic Sea Salt or Himalayan Salt
* 2 TBSP Vanilla Extract
* 2 pasture raised eggs or egg substitute (pg 155 & 231)
* 2 cups (12 oz) unsweetened dark chocolate cacao nibs
  (or make your own chocolate or carob chips)

Helpful Tip: Look at the original directions and know that the first time you make this recipe, it may need some alterations. When I first make a recipe with multiple ingredients, I make a very small batch. Start by cutting the batch by one-quarter or one-half -- whatever works best for the recipe. Another option is to bake just a few and then taste test. Does the recipe need more sweetness, salt or flour? Then adjust accordingly to taste/flavor and texture.

Directions:

1. Preheat oven to 350. In a bowl, mix dry ingredients together (except chocolate chips).
2. In a DIFFERENT bowl, mix the wet ingredients together.
3. Slowly fold dry ingredients into the wet ingredients and mix well.
4. Add in chocolate chips and gently mix into batter.
5. Use a glass baking container or stainless steel baking sheet. Grease container/sheet with coconut oil or organic butter or Ghee, or line with natural parchment paper. You can use a tablespoon or your favorite dough utensil to scoop out to desired size.
6. Bake until edges are golden and the center is soft. Depending on your oven and size of the cookies, bake 8-10 minutes. Remove from oven and cool before eating. Store cookies in an air-tight container for about a week (if they last that long).

❋ Upgrade: Switch all ingredients to organic

Instead of regular pastry flour --> Upgrade to Organic Whole Grain Flour.
Instead of Refined Sugar --> Organic Coconut Sugar. (**See Upgraded Sweeteners pg 83**)

❋ Upgrade: Take regular cookie recipe and Upgrade the ingredients. See Recipe above.
Refer to Upgrade chart and choose the most nourishing ingredients.

❋ Upgrade: Vegans - Substitute butter and eggs. (**See Conversions on the next page**)

Examples of Upgrades (Vegan Friendly)

Old Item	UPGRADED Item
Butter (fake butters)	Organic Extra Virgin Coconut Oil or Organic Extra Virgin Olive Oil
Eggs (binders/gums)	Flax Seeds or Chia Seeds
Dairy (soy milk etc.)	Nut or Seed Milks, Coconut Butter, Coconut or Olive oil
Cream (soy)	Avocado, Coconut Butter, Oil or Coconut Cream or Cashew Cream

Ingredient Conversions

When you see the term one to one (1:1) It means swap out the original amount for exactly the same amount. For example: If the original recipe calls for 1 cup flour, swap out 1 cup almond flour in the upgraded recipe.

Flour

If the recipe calls for white flour and you want that gooey consistency and do fine with gluten: Swap organic whole wheat flour for the white flour 1:1.

Using BEANS instead of flour
* Swap 1 cup of flour for 1 cup of bean puree
* Black beans, kidney beans, mung beans, and adzuki beans work great. Find your favorite taste and swap for flour.

Coconut Flour
Recipe calls for 2 cups of wheat flour – upgrade to the following:
* 1 cup Gluten-free grain
* 1 Cup Coconut flour
* 1 ADDITIONAL cup of liquids
* Double the egg or flax slurry

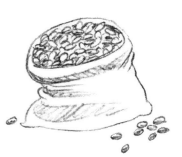

1 cup Wheat flour = 1/3 cup coconut flour + DOUBLE the eggs + MORE water/milk

Coconut flour is very absorbent.
* First, check the consistency of the 'dough' and then take notes so you can make it easier the next time. Mix coconut flour more than regular flour because it easily clumps.
* Use LESS coconut flour than what a recipe calls for (because of its absorbency).

Baking with Coconut Flour: It usually takes **LESS time to bake** with coconut flour than wheat flour:
* 30 minutes for Wheat flour = Approx. 15-20 minutes for Coconut flour
* 50 minutes for Wheat flour = Approx. 20-25 minutes for Coconut flour

For almond flour or other nut flours
* Swap 1 cup of flour for 1 cup of bean puree
* Black beans, kidney beans, mung beans, and adzuki beans work great.

Flour Tips:
* If you are not ready to go full on with switching over to flour or beans. Then start adding in some flour or beans into the recipe, and then slowly decrease the amount of whole wheat flour… just to ease in a little.
* Remember non-glutenous flours and beans will not make it stick like glue as the GLUEten-ous flours.
* Nut flours will not rise like regular flour so take that into account.

Baking Powder

Usually derived from GMO cornstarch. If a recipe calls for baking powder, you can use this instead:

Old	UPGRADED
1 tsp of baking powder	1-1/2 tsp lemon juice or apple cider vinegar & 1/4 tsp baking **soda** (aluminum FREE)

Butter Butter, Butter!

Old	UPGRADED
Toxic Margarine Toxic Fake Butters	Organic Grass-Fed Butter Organic Grass-Fed Ghee

For *Vegans or Dairy Intolerant, here are some excellent **BUTTER alternatives**:

Old	UPGRADED
Regular Butter or Toxic Fake Butters Margarines	Avocado puree * One to one - it takes a little getting used to, but give it a whirl Banana functions similar to avocado * For fats, use avocado (above) * For a sweeter taste, use banana * Use 1 cup mashed banana instead of 1cup of oil Prunes * In brownies and darker baked goods * Soak prunes in water and then puree * One to one Chia seeds for butter * 1 TBSP butter for 9 TBSP water * Sit 15 minutes and allow to gel, stir often Coconut Oil or Coconut Butter * One to one Nut Butter * One to one

Old	UPGRADED
Margarine Fake Butter Spreads	Butter, Ghee, Coconut Oil or Pasture Raised Animal Fat * One to one
Peanut Butter (Hydrogenated/sugar etc.)	Almond butter (or other Organic & plain nut/seed butters) * One to one
Hydrogenated Oils Canola/Vegetable Oils Soy Oil	Coconut Oil, Organic Grass-Fed Butter, Organic Ghee, Pasture Raised Animal Fat * One to one
Sugary Chocolate	Cacao nibs Raw cacao powder or cacao butter Organic unsweetened chocolate chips (check ingredients) *May need to INCREASE Sweetener if recipe calls for sweetened chocolate. Make your own chocolate chips * (cacao powder, cacao butter, coconut sugar)

Refined Sugar Upgrades

Unsweetened applesauce

* Swap applesauce for sugar one to one
* Make your own applesauce if possible, or find an organic version without any additives.
* **You may need to reduce other liquids by 1/4 cup for every cup of applesauce used.** If you want it sweeter, ease up on other liquids.

Banana

* Swap banana for sugar one to one
* Use as your base for Ice Cream - replaces dairy and sweetener

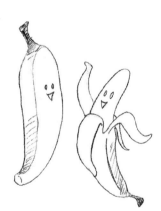

Vanilla

* Use 1/2 teaspoon of vanilla for every 2 TBSP of sugar that you replace.
* Be sure to use organic vanilla. Caution: many generic vanilla extracts are made with corn syrup or other undesirables.

Raw Honey

* Swap honey for sugar or other syrups one to one
* I tend to use honey in its raw state for desserts that do not need to be cooked.

Stevia

* 1 tsp liquid stevia or 1 tsp stevia powder for 1 cup of sugar
* Swap any artificial sweeteners for organic stevia.

See Sugar/Upgraded Sweeteners in Chapter 4, pages 77, 83-85 for more options.

Eggs

Old	UPGRADED
Regular Eggs	Organic, NON-GMO feed, No Antibiotics or Hormones Pasture Raised Eggs
Egg Replacer Any egg-stuff in a carton, powder etc.	Chia seeds for eggs Use this for each egg you replace * 1 TBSP chia with 1 cup water * Sit to gel and stir Flax eggs Substitute this for 1 egg * 1 TBSP ground flax seeds (flax meal) * 3 TBSP warm water * Whisk to combine * Sit in fridge 5-10 minutes

Thickeners

Old	UPGRADED
Fake Thickeners Gums	* Chia Seeds * Flax Seeds * Coconut Oil/Butter * Avocado * **Arrowroot** * **Kuzu** * **Agar Agar** *** Check instructions on packages for thickening conversions**

Dairy

Old	UPGRADED
Regular Dairy	Organic Pasture Raised, Grass-Fed, Hormone and Antibiotic Free Dairy
Vegan Non-Dairy Products (milk, cream, yogurt, etc.)	Coconut Milk or Coconut Cream Organic Sheep or Goat products
Artificial or Sugar Based Non-Dairy Products	Coconut Butter/Oil/Milk/Cream Nuts or Seed Butters

FAST Carb Conversions

Old	UPGRADED
White Rice	Brown Rice
Couscous	Quinoa
Pasta	Thin Zucchini slices - spiralized or julienned. Can be raw, lightly steamed, or sautéed Spaghetti Squash, Brown Rice, or Quinoa Pasta
Potato	Cauliflower, turnip, sweet potato, celery root: Almost any mashed root vegetable can replace white potatoes for mashed potatoes
Bread Crumbs	Baked Rolled Oats, Homemade Granola, Nutrtional Yeast or Ground Flax Seeds
Tortilla	NON-GMO Corn, Sprouted Whole Grain Tortillas, Lettuce Leaves, or Collard Greens
French Fries	Homemade with Organic Potatoes or Sweet Potatoes
Candy/Pastries	Organic, Upgraded ingredients or homemade

The Sticky on Gums a.k.a. - Binders

There are quite a few binders out there which are used extensively in gluten-free baking. For someone with digestive issues, I don't recommend this. Do your research and taste test. Remember that what may be poison for one person could be medicine to another. If you are not comfortable using the gums (i.e. xanthan gum, guar gum, etc.), use flax or chia seeds instead. These create a similar gummy texture (the thing in gluten that holds everything together).

A few examples:

* Cellulose Gum
* Guar Gum
* Tara Gum
* Gellan Gum
* Gum Arabic
* Xanthan Gum

*Not a complete list. **Many binders DO NOT have the word 'gum' in them.** When in doubt, research the positive AND negative of an ingredient and decide for yourself.

Be patient with your creations. First, make sure it tastes really great and then work on the texture. If the texture is good but the taste isn't, you are more likely to trash it than if the texture is a little off, but tastes really good. It's a great idea to bake or cook a small portion to see if it agrees with your taste buds. If needed, alter the recipe and make notes as you go. Use an index card holder or notebook to create a personal cookbook.

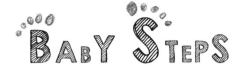

Create your favorite sauce from scratch or find an organic version in the store.

Alter the recipe of your favorite sweet treat or snack food, and create an Upgraded version.

Start by altering recipes of your favorite meals. Get creative and search online or in healthy cookbooks for more ideas. Create your own recipe catalogue for easy access. See Recipe section.

Portion Control?

Forgettabout it!!! Seriously, think about it: eating anything in sight when you feel you're being 'bad' to thinking that 'good' means eating healthy food AND controlling portions. You go from one extreme to the other -- stuffing your face to near starvation. This is the reason why diets don't work. When you begin to Upgrade your foods and eat nourishing and natural foods, you need to eat enough to feel satisfied. Eating until you are satisfied keeps you invested in the Upgrade process. Portion control will harmonize itself naturally. Have you ever binged uncontrollably on broccoli? At first, allow yourself to eat more than you 'think you should'. You probably need to eat more at first in order to feel satisfied enough for the Upgrade process to really work for you.

How to Upgrade Your Family & Get Them on Board

Do you have to feed your family as well? Make a slow transition so the whole process goes smoothly. First, find all of the condiments that your family loves and place them in the center of the table. Family -style meals can be a lot of fun if you have a turn table (Lazy Susan) in the center of the table for easy access. I had a friend named Susan who hated the fact that this gadget was called a Lazy Susan. Since then I think of her and call them turn tables instead.

Kids will love this process, especially if you involve them. Allow your family to serve and sauce their own food. This cuts down on the amount of time spent cooking for five different picky eaters and their taste buds. Next is a sample food plan you can use to create family-style meals.

If you are vegan or vegetarian, please don't be offended that I included meat suggestions here. If you eat meat/dairy, you don't have to go vegan. As I mentioned in the beginning of this book, only YOU and your body know what's best for you. Your family's needs are different than your neighbor's down the street. I give you a variety of options so you can choose what works well for you and your family. Your family's food plan can include a variety of possibilities as long as your family follows the Upgrade concept of clean, real, and nutrient-packed foods.

Breakfast Options

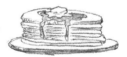

Make Your Own Yogurt Combination:
* Yogurt
* Berries
* Ground Flax Seeds
* Nuts and Seeds / Homemade Granola

Instead of Cereal:
* Whole Grains: Quinoa, Brown Rice, Gluten-Free Oats, Gluten-Free Steel Cut Oats
* Berries, Fresh or Dried Fruit (Organic Raisins, Dates and/or Goji Berries)
* Organic Grass Fed, Plain Cow/Goat/Sheep Yogurt (add your own toppings)
* Flax Seeds, Chia Seeds or any other Nut/Seed or Nut/Seed Butters
* Token Vegetable (i.e. Steamed Kale, Steamed Carrots, or Collard Greens)

If you/your family are sausage, bacon, eggs, and potato breakfast people:
* Find the best quality ingredients
* Sausage and Bacon: No hormones, no nitrates, organic/NON-GMO feed
* Pasture Raised Eggs (NON-GMO feed, soy and corn-free if possible)

Potatoes:
* Organic roasted, boiled, baked or fried in Coconut Oil
* Try sweet potatoes or upgrade to Quinoa, Brown Rice, or Gluten-Free Oats

Pancakes:
* Whole Grains and Upgraded Sweeteners. Upgrade with the conversion charts.

Smoothie/ Protein Powder
* Many smoothie and protein powders contain yucky ingredients so it's better to make your own. Why? When you strip down ingredients, it strips down the taste. Taste and texture make food palatable. So they have to add in some undesirables to make it desirable.

Morning Smoothie Options
* If Whey gives you energy and protein, find Organic, NON-GMO, Grass Fed Whey.
* Create a smoothie bar. If your mornings are busy, buy all your ingredients separately and then combine them into a container, so it's just a one scoop job.

See Recipe Section for more ideas.

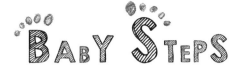

BABY STEPS

1 **Highlight or make note of the foods listed in this chapter that you are interested in trying:**

2 **Out of the items you highlighted, which ones do you want to try this week?**

3 **After you try any of the items you highlighted, go back and put a check mark next to the ones you enjoyed, and cross out the ones that didn't appeal to you.** This helps when you go back to reference. You will immediately know which new items you want to try, which ones you enjoyed, and which ones you don't need to bother with again.

Note: If you think something is 'good for you' but you don't enjoy it – then it's that 'diet mentality' you want to Upgrade from. Enjoy the foods you eat!

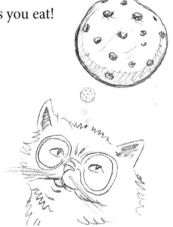

In Chapter 6, we discussed:
* The heart of Upgradeology
* Easy Upgrades to get you started
* Food to Upgrade from and why
* Upgrades for everything from Meals to Snacks
* Upgrading your Condiments and Beverages
* The reality of Caffeine and your cleanest sources
* How to alter and Upgrade recipes
* Cooking and Baking conversions
* Why there are so many gums and binders in the foods
* Why letting go of portion control is essential when beginning the Upgrading process
* Getting family and friends on board

The Food and Beverage Upgrades discussed in this chapter show you how to Upgrade from Frankenfoods! You learned many ways to begin incorporating Upgrades for the foods you love. Be sure to come back to this chapter as a reference when baking, cooking, or when looking for delicious Upgraded ideas. This chapter was packed with a LOT of ideas on how to convert recipes so you can still indulge in your favorite foods!

Let's keep going with Healing Foods. In the next chapter, you will discover many of the beneficial nutrients of the foods contained within this book.

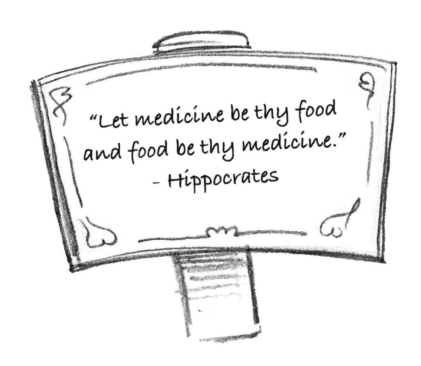

7.Healingology

Learn How to Increase Energy With Nourishing Foods

Index of Healing Foods

The Healing Foods listed below (not a complete list) give you a quick reference of the nutrient-dense foods discussed throughout the previous chapters. Many of these foods can help alleviate health issues caused by the refined, artificial and processed foods you are now learning to Upgrade. This chapter is another reminder to transition towards eating clean, nourishing, and real organic foods whenever possible.

Acai

Benefits: Acai is rich in antioxidants, an immune-stimulating and energy-boosting berry. It is packed with nutrients and is the exotic version of a blueberry or cranberry.

Uses: Acai can be found in many forms. Use organic Acai in smoothies and homemade protein shakes. Add into homemade yogurt or ice cream.

Almond Flour

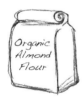

Benefits: Almond flour is full of fiber, protein and magnesium. It is gluten-free and has a lower glycemic index than traditional flours.

Uses: Since it's denser than traditional flours, research before replacing in recipes (See recipe conversions on page 152) Great for pancakes and baked goods!

Almonds

Benefits: Full of fiber, magnesium and calcium. Provides a quick energy boost!

Uses: Almonds can be made into almond milk and added to nut mixes. Available in nut butters (use instead of peanut butter). Chop them up and use them in salads, or sprinkle on top of soups. Almonds are an easy, energy efficient snack. These make a great night snack because they are full of magnesium and are a calming food.

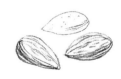

Aloe Vera

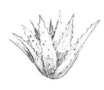

Benefits: A powerful and soothing digestive aide. Stabilizes blood sugar and is full of enzymes, vitamins and minerals.

Uses: Excellent to use directly on the skin for first aid needs such as cuts, sores and especially burns. Best to use from the Aloe Vera plant, they are easy to grow and maintain.

Amaranth

Benefits: Amaranth is an ancient grain filled with protein and calcium. Since it is gluten-free, people with Celiac disease can eat it without worry. Has a delicious corn-like flavor.

Uses: It can be used in place of other grains in recipes (i.e. tabouli). It also makes a delicious, hot morning breakfast cereal. You can even pop it like mini-mini popcorn.

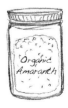

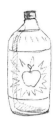

Apple Cider Vinegar, RAW & Organic

Benefits: Is anti-viral, anti-bacterial, and anti-fungal! It's full of potassium and helps balance your body's pH levels. It's an excellent digestive aide and overall health tonic.

Uses: Upgrade all of your vinegars to Apple Cider Vinegar. Great for salad dressings and vinegar-based foods. Has a plethora of uses. (See Add-Ins page 31)

Apples

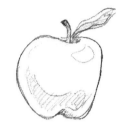

Benefits: Apples are full of fiber, antioxidants, and a great source of B complex Vitamins. They are a great source of energy without the caffeine jitters!

Uses: Make your own low-sugar applesauce or add apples to salads! They taste delicious with almond butter as an energy snack and are extremely portable.

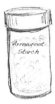

Arrowroot Starch

Benefits: It's easy to digest and even safe for infants! It's gluten-free and aids in digestion. It can act as mild laxative for those who struggle with digestive issues.

Uses: Makes a great thickener for stews, sauces, and pie fillings (a great alternative to cornstarch). It can also be added to gluten-free baked goods to make the density lighter.

Asparagus

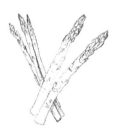

Benefits: This green veggie is full of anti-oxidants and decreases inflammation. It contains a great deal of folate, Vitamin K, and Vitamin C.

Uses: A delicious vegetable that can be eaten steamed or roasted. Drizzle with olive oil and apple cider vinegar to pack in flavor. Sauté fresh strawberries to put over the top!

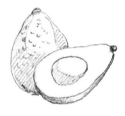

Avocados

Benefits: Avocados are a great source of Vitamin E with 25 essential nutrients - more than double the potassium found in bananas.

Uses: These are great by themselves, or mashed up for guacamole. Use in a smoothie to replace dairy. Mix with cacao powder and an Upgraded Sweetener to create pudding.

Bananas

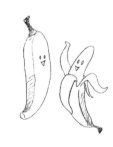

Benefits: Bananas contains high levels of tryptophan, which can help alleviate some depression. They help improve the immune system, and are full of fiber and potassium.

Uses: Freeze and then blend them to make a delicious ice cream-like dessert! They're also a great snack and breakfast topper for homemade granola, whole grains, and porridge.

Basil

Benefits: Basil contains a high amount of Vitamin K and calcium. It acts as an anti-inflammatory, anti-oxidant and anti-bacterial. Basil also aids with digestion.

Uses: For the best results, use fresh, organic leaves. Basil can be added to most meals for flavorful health benefits.

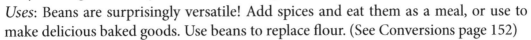

Beans

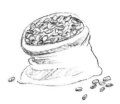

Benefits: Beans are very high in fiber, but also contain iron and lots of antioxidants. They also regulate how your blood absorbs glucose.

Uses: Beans are surprisingly versatile! Add spices and eat them as a meal, or use to make delicious baked goods. Use beans to replace flour. (See Conversions page 152)

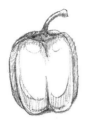

Bell Peppers

Benefits: Bell Peppers are full of Vitamin C, potassium and fiber. They are an antioxidant, can reduce inflammation, and regulate blood pressure.

Uses: These are delicious in salads, or sauté them and add to soups and stews! The variety of colors add life and beauty to the foods you add them to.

Blueberries

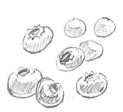

Benefits: These blue gems are full of Vitamin C, fiber and high in antioxidants. Blueberries help boost your immune system, improve memory, and increase brain health!

Uses: They make a great snack on their own, or can be added to a variety of dishes. Blueberries taste excellent in smoothies or as a breakfast topper.

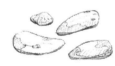

Brazil Nuts

Benefits: An excellent source of selenium, magnesium, phosphorus and thiamine. They also contain zinc, copper and Vitamin E. They contain 'heart-healthy' fats.

Uses: Just a few per day will provide you with a healthy dose of selenium. Add to nut mixes, sprinkle on vegetables, salads or soups.

Broccoli

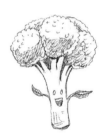

Benefits: Broccoli is full of antioxidants, beta-carotene, and has more calcium than most dairy products! It helps regulate blood sugar and blood pressure.

Uses: Broccoli is a great veggie to add to your stews, soups, and sauces! You can even blend it into sauces to increase its nutritional value.

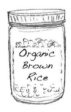

Brown Rice (Sprouted)

Benefits: Sprouted brown rice has many health benefits compared to other rice. It is gluten-free and has seven times more magnesium and fiber than regular rice.

Uses: You can eat brown rice in so many different ways. Makes a delicious gluten-free risotto, use leftovers for morning porridge or to replace flour in cookies.

Basmati Brown Rice

Benefits: Tends to cook quicker than Brown Rice. Thinner and longer than brown rice. Full of nutrients, flavor and aroma.

Uses: Commonly used in Indian Cooking. An excellent aromatic Gluten-Free Whole Grain. Use instead of brown rice to flavor up a dish.

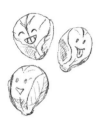

Brussels Sprouts

Benefits: Brussels sprouts are high in antioxidants and Vitamin C! Its dietary fiber can help control and lower harmful cholesterol.

Uses: Makes a beautiful side dish. Slice and cook just until they are done, or roast them with your favorite spices. Make them taste delicious to you!

Buckwheat Flour

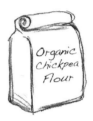

Benefits: Buckwheat is gluten-free (with low allergens) and full of essential nutrients.

Uses: Its nutty flavor makes it a great option for pancakes and baked goods. Substitute 100% buckwheat Soba Noodles for other pasta. Read ingredients carefully because most 'soba' noodles are mostly whole wheat.

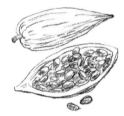

Buckwheat Grouts

Benefits: Buckwheat grouts are full of rutin. They are good for capillaries, decrease blood pressure, and can increase circulation in extremities.

Uses: Another name is Kasha (don't confuse with the brand name). They can be lightly toasted and eaten plain, or add to other veggies for a nice salad.

Burdock

Benefits: Burdock has healing benefits for the skin and is used to purify the blood. It's also a diuretic and can assist eliminating the body of harmful toxins.

Uses: Burdock can be peeled, sliced and added to soups or stews. The root can be brewed as a tea and blood purifying tonic.

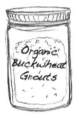

Cacao

Benefits: Full of protein, calcium, magnesium, copper, zinc, iron and antioxidants. Contains phenethylamine, a chemical compound sometimes called the "love chemical."

Uses: Add to baked goods and other dishes to create a full-bodied flavor. Use with your favorite sweetener to replace sugary chocolate.

Cacao Butter, Cacao Paste & Cacao Powder

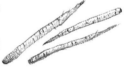

Benefits: Cacao butter and cacao paste can be melted down for your chocolate base. They create that smooth 'chocolate bar' texture.

Uses: Organic Cacao Powder replaces any chocolate powder in your recipes. Make your own hot cocoa or homemade mocha. (See Add-Ins page 30).

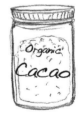

Cacao Nibs

Benefits: Cacao Nibs are bitter, not sweet, but they add a nice flavor to replace chocolate in recipes. You may need to increase Upgraded sweeteners when these are used.

Uses: These are for all the dark chocolate lovers out there. Add a few to trail mixes. Use to replace chocolate chips in baked goods.

Cardamom

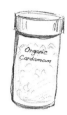

Benefits: Is an excellent digestive aide and anti-inflammatory. It can assist easing nausea, bloating, gas and heartburn. Ayurvedic's suggest that it can ease depression too.

Uses: Cardamom is a unique spice, often added to curry powders. Add it to sweet foods for balance (see Almond Cardamom Cookies). It is a main ingredient in Garam Masala.

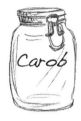

Carob Powder

Benefits: It is a good source of calcium - includes other essential vitamins and minerals. An excellent caffeine free alternative for chocolate.

Uses: Carob has a strong sweet flavor and makes a good substitute for chocolate. Mix with yogurt or avocado to make a pudding! Use instead of chocolate for hot drinks.

Carrots

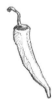

Benefits: Carrots help improve your eye sight and may prevent heart disease. They are full of antioxidants and Vitamin K. Eating carrots can flush toxins from your body.

Uses: Carrots are another easy snack - eat with your favorite dip. They can be shredded and added to recipes. Carrots can also be steamed or boiled (makes a sweet puree).

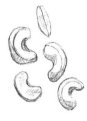

Cashews

Benefits: Cashews are packed with dietary fiber and healthy monounsaturated fatty acids. They provide magnesium, copper, and other minerals.

Uses: Enjoy these as part of a trail mix or alone. Put them through a food processor to make a great nut butter! For a whipped topping, soak in water for an hour, then blend.

Cauliflower

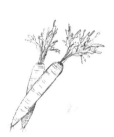

Benefits: One cup of cauliflower provides you with potassium, Vitamin C, and fiber! It's an antioxidant with anti-inflammatory properties.

Uses: Cauliflower is extremely versatile. Chop it and eat raw, steam it, bake it, boil or sauté. It can be steamed and mashed up to make mock mashed potatoes.

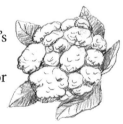

Cayenne Pepper

Benefits: Cayenne pepper increases metabolic rate and stimulates the circulatory system. Excellent to add flavor and spice your food.

Uses: Use as an anti-inflammatory (especially good for arthritis sufferers). Add cayenne pepper to your food to give it a spicy kick!

Celeriac or Celery Root

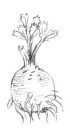

Benefits: Celeriac is a great source of Vitamin K, phosphorous, iron, calcium and magnesium. Excellent to aid in digestive issues and stimulate metabolism.

Uses: Its flavor is an earthy version of celery. Use as an alternative to mashed potatoes, or bake them like fries. You can also shred it, or use it in the same way you would a potato.

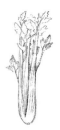

Celery

Benefits: Celery is an alkalizing food that helps reduce blood pressure and lower cholesterol. It can improve the health of your immune system too. It's an energizing food!

Uses: Because of its salty flavor, it acts like a flavor binder. It adds dimension to soups & stews. Celery, carrot, and onion create the essential ingredients to start a soup stock.

Celtic Sea Salt

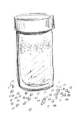

Benefits: Celtic Sea Salt contains essential trace minerals and powerful electrolytes such as magnesium. Helps prevent cramping and balances blood sugar levels.

Uses: Add to food to bring out it's natural flavor. Replace other salts, including regular sea salt and table salts. Beneficial in diabetic cooking.

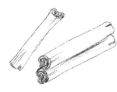

Ceylon Cinnamon

Benefits: Ceylon Added to your food can help control blood sugar. It has anti-inflammatory properties, contains manganese and iron and may help reduce migraine headaches.

Uses: Cinnamon is a flavorful spice. Add to your morning cereals, baked goods, and warm drinks. See Add-Ins on page 28.

Cherries

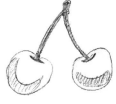

Benefits: Out of all the fruits, cherries contain some of the highest levels of beta-carotenes. They are high in antioxidants, anti-cancer agents, and phytonutrients.

Uses: Enjoy fresh, organic cherries when they are in season. They are delicious in smoothies or eat as a frozen treat in hot temperatures.

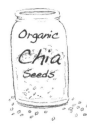

Chia Seed

Benefits: Chia seeds are full of protein, fiber, vitamins and minerals. Chia seeds absorb the water they are soaked in and help to retain electrolytes and keep you hydrated.

Uses: Add to your favorite nut milk to make a breakfast pudding. Add to smoothies for additional protein and fiber benefits. Can be sprouted and added to salads. See Add-Ins.

Chickpeas

Benefits: Chickpeas can assist with blood sugar regulation. They are high in fiber, protein and nutrients. A beneficial food for diabetics.

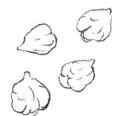

Uses: Blend chickpeas with garlic and other spices to create a fiber-filled hummus! These can be added to soups and salads too.

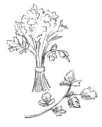

Cilantro

Benefits: It helps to remove toxins from your body and is full of antioxidants. Cilantro encourages liver function and helps control blood sugar.

Uses: Cilantro makes a great garnish for salads, or add to your homemade salsa or smoothies. Dried cilantro adds flavor cooking soups or stews.

Coconut Crystals (Raw) / Coconut Sugar / Coconut Palm Sugar

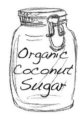

Benefits: Coconut crystals / sugar are a low glycemic, gluten-free food that contain fiber, 17 amino acids, minerals and vitamins (including B Vitamins).

Uses: Replace one to one with other sugars. This is the most recommended sweetener, besides organic green leaf stevia, for diabetics and those with blood sugar issues.

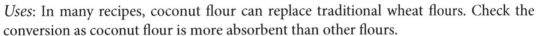

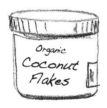

Coconut Flakes

Benefits: Coconut flakes are a great source of medium-chain fatty acids, lauric acid, manganese, and iron. They are high in dietary fiber and can help lower cholesterol.

Uses: Bake coconut flakes to make a crunchy and delicious snack. Use in raw desserts, or add to your homemade trail mix or granola bars.

Coconut Flour

Benefits: It's gluten-free and good for blood sugar stabilization. Coconut flour has more than 50% of the dietary fiber found in other flours!

Uses: In many recipes, coconut flour can replace traditional wheat flours. Check the conversion as coconut flour is more absorbent than other flours.

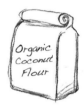

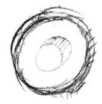

Coconut Milk

Benefits: Coconut milk is the only source (other than breast milk) that contains lauric acid. Lauric acid prevents fungus growth, inhibits viruses, and is an anti-microbial.

Uses: Replace regular milk or creamers with coconut milk. Tastes delicious in beverages or use in Thai based soups and curries! Used extensively with vegans and raw foodies.

Coconut Nectar

Benefits: It is a low glycemic sweetener. Coconut nectar contains amino acids, minerals, and Vitamin C and B!

Uses: Add to beverages as a natural sweetener. Drizzle on pancakes like maple syrup, and use one to one for other liquid sweeteners in recipes.

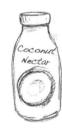

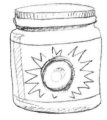

Coconut Oil

Benefits: Coconut oil is full of medium chain fatty acids. It can assist with blood sugar stabilization, help increase metabolism, and assist with weight release.

Uses: Coconut Oil is an ideal replacement for other toxic cooking oils. Can be used to replace diary in recipes. Is an excellent skin moisturizer and healer.

Cucumbers

Benefits: Cucumbers are a great source of Vitamin B and C! These help your body remove toxins and improve joint health.

Uses: Cucumbers taste great raw. They are heavy in water content and can even be used in smoothies. Place them in apple cider vinegar to pickle them.

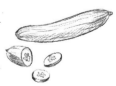

Daikon Radish

Benefits: Contains enzymes that aid in fat and starch digestion. Contains high levels of Vitamin C, phosphorous and potassium. Contains phyto-nutrients that are anti-cancer. Often used in Asian cuisine. Use in stir frys, shred and add to salads or ferment and use as a digestive aide. You can also juice it or cut it up and brew it like a tea.

Dandelion Greens

Benefits: One cup contains more than 100% of your daily intake of Vitamin A. These greens are full of calcium and iron! They are a natural diuretic and help clean the blood.
Uses: Dandelion greens can be eaten raw, steamed, or even blended. They have a pleasant pungent-ness to them and add variety to salads and vegetable dishes.

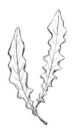

Dill

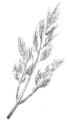

Benefits: Dill is an excellent source of calcium, manganese, and iron. It helps with digestion and flushes out toxins. Dill is also an antioxidant and anti-bacterial.
Uses: Dill is a very easy to use spice. Use fresh, organic dill whenever you can. It's great in salad greens, soups, and stews.

Dulse Flakes

Benefits: Dulse flakes are full of trace minerals and phytonutrients, and support the immune and nervous system.
Uses: Replace bacon with crunchy dulse on sandwiches and salads. Grind it up for a delicious addition to your soup or salad!

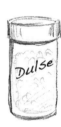

Flaxseed (ground)

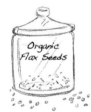

Benefits: There are almost too many to list! Flaxseed helps protect your bones, and helps prevent cancer and regulates cholesterol. It also helps increase insulin response.
Uses: Mix flaxseed into your morning breakfast cereal or add to a smoothie. It can also be added to a variety of baked goods.

Garam Masala

Benefits: Garam Masala means "hot mixture." A a blend of ground spices that usually contain: peppercorns, cloves, mace, cumin, cardamom, nutmeg, anise, and coriander.
Uses: It's a delightful mixture that you can buy pre-mixed or make your own. Use it for curry dishes, and makes an excellent pairing with lentils too.

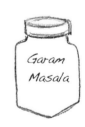

Garbanzo Bean Flour (Chickpeas)

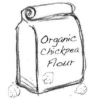

Benefits: Garbanzo bean flour is high in protein and fiber. It's gluten-free and extremely versatile in baking and cooking.
Uses: Add it to other flours to make them more nutritious. It can also be used to make pizzas, thicken soups, and other dishes that you would normally use flour.

Garlic

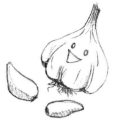

Benefits: Garlic helps manage blood sugar levels and lower high blood pressure. It's anti-viral and anti-parasitic.

Uses: Add garlic to all sorts of foods in your everyday meal planning. It's also beneficial to consume when you feel under the weather.

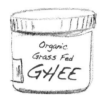

Ghee

Benefits: Ghee is lactose and casein free. It also assists with digestion and absorption of nutrients. An excellent alternative for those who are dairy sensitive.

Uses: Since it's clarified butter, it can be used in the exact same way as butter. It has a higher heat tolerance than other oils, and can be used to sauté foods.

Ginger

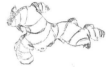

Benefits: Ginger can alleviate digestive discomfort and boosts your immune system. It's anti-fungal, anti-bacterial, and anti-viral.

Uses: Tastes great in curries and other foods, but is especially beneficial when you feel sick. Shred some fresh ginger root into hot water to make an immune boosting tea.

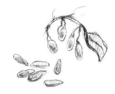

Goji Berries

Benefits: Goji berries are full of antioxidants. They help balance blood sugar, and assist with liver function and digestion.

Uses: Goji berries are great in smoothies, granola bars, and trail mix. Grind them up and mold them into a delicious candy!

Grapefruit

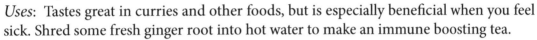

Benefits: Grapefruit is full of Vitamin C and is an immune-boosting, low glycemic fruit. Contains anti-inflammatory properties that can assist easing joint pain and arthritis.

Uses: Slice and eat as a refreshing snack. Juice them and add to salad dressings for zing.

Warning: Check with your Dr. if you are on any medications before eating grapefruit.

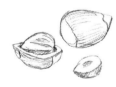

Hazelnuts

Benefits: These nuts are full of Vitamin E, and Vitamins B1, B3, B5, B6, and B9. Hazelnuts also contain manganese and copper, and are rich in unsaturated fats!

Uses: Grind hazelnuts to make nut butter, or add to baked goods to boost their nutritional values. Delicious in snack mixes and granola bars.

Hemp Seeds

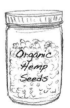

Benefits: Hemp seeds contain high levels of magnesium, iron, zinc, and fiber! These seeds are also full of protein, essential amino acids, and beneficial fats.

Uses: Sprinkle on favorite foods, or use in smoothies and granola bars. Adds a mild nutty flavor to foods. Add to fruits to slow down the natural sugar assimilation.

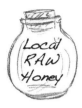

Honey, Raw & Unprocessed (Local if possible)

Benefits: Raw honey is full of Vitamins C and B, and polyphenols. Eat local raw honey to help with seasonal allergies and increase immune strength.

Uses: Replace other liquid sweeteners with honey or add some to your tea! Use to replace corn syrup, agave or other sugars in recipes.

Horseradish Root

Benefits: This root has long been used in "folk remedies". It's full of glucosinolates which help with sinus and other respiratory issues. It's also full of vitamin C!

Uses: Its sharp, hot flavor is a great addition to different foods. Horseradish root tastes great when made into a spicy cream sauce.

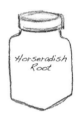

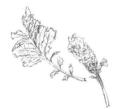

Kale

Benefits: Kale is a leafy green vegetable with many benefits! It's high in iron, antioxidants, and calcium. It also helps detoxify your body!

Uses: Kales make a delicious chip! Toss lightly in coconut oil and sea salt before baking. They also taste delicious in "massaged" salads.

Kelp

Benefits: Kelp is full of iodine, and Vitamin A, D, E, and K. Kelp has that umami flavor to it and is an excellent natural flavor enhancer.

Uses: Eat with the seasoning of your choice, or add to soups and stews to increase the nutrition. Can be used instead of salt.

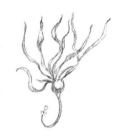

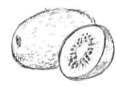

Kiwi

Benefits: Kiwi contains more Vitamin C than oranges! It's also a great source of fiber, iron, and calcium!

Uses: Add sliced kiwi to a fruit salad. In season, they are refreshing and cooling in a smoothie.

Lemons

Benefits: Lemons are very alkaline and act as a blood purifier. They also help balance blood sugar and have anti-bacterial properties.

Uses: Add lemon to your water to help boost your immune and digestive system. Add to salad dressings or just squeeze on top of salads.

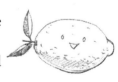

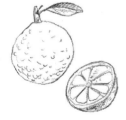

Limes

Benefits: Limes help digest food and burn fat, and have even more Vitamin C than lemons!

Uses: Add limes to your water, or juice on top of fruits for extra flavor. Used in guacamole and often with corn dishes.

Lucuma

Benefits: Lucuma is a fantastic source of fiber, Vitamin B3, Iron, and beta-carotene.

Uses: This lightly sweet powder can be added to foods that need sweetness (i.e. puddings, ice creams, smoothies, and breakfast meals). It's very subtle and not as sweet as most sweeteners.

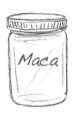

Maca Powder

Benefits: Maca powder helps balance hormones, and is full of protein and seven essential amino acids. It can also help manage depression and increase memory.

Uses: Add maca powder to smoothies, hot chocolate, coffee/tea drinks or with the Golden Milk Recipe. You can also use it in Horchata. See recipe section.

Macadamia Nuts

Benefits: These nuts are rich in fiber and are a natural antioxidant. They're high in mono-unsaturated fats, protein, and essential amino acids (a great boost for brain function).

Uses: Macadamia nuts are full of flavor. Add to trail mix and other snacks.

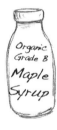

Maple Syrup

Benefits: Maple syrup contains manganese and zinc, and high levels of calcium and potassium. It acts as an antioxidant and can decrease inflammation.

Uses: Maple syrup is a great way to add natural sweetness to different dishes.

Matcha Green Tea Powder

Benefits: Matcha green tea (like most organic green teas) is full of antioxidants, and a cleaner form of caffeine. It is an energy booster yet it's calming without the usual jitters from coffee or caffeinated drinks. It's a stable alternative for blood sugar issues.

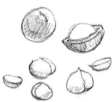

Uses: You can create a delicious warm green tea drink out of it. Add it to smoothies. You can even add it to frozen bananas and create an 'ice cream' out of it.

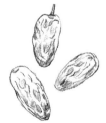

Medjool Dates

Benefits: Medjool dates are high in iron, potassium, and dietary fiber. These are an excellent source of vegan protein. As a snack, they are a great source of energy!

Uses: Use as an alternative sweetener to sugar! Soak dates and then grind them down to create a delicious syrup or paste.

Mesquite Powder

Benefits: Mesquite powder is a great source of nutrients including protein. It also contains minerals including calcium and magnesium. It is low in the glycemic index.

Uses: Mesquite powder has a sweet caramel flavor and makes a great addition to smoothies. Note: the powder does not taste like mesquite barbeque.

Miso Paste

Benefits: There are almost too many to list! It's a complete protein which means it has all of the essential amino acids. It's a digestive aide (a probiotic). Excellent source of B12 and other B vitamins (is an antioxidant). May help protect against radiation from the environment, and reduce the risk of cancer. It helps balance cholesterol, and boosts your immune system. Use in soups, dressings and sauces. See page 123.

Mushrooms

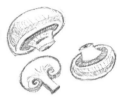

Benefits: Extremely important to get Organic or Wild mushrooms. Organic mushrooms can assist with healthy immune function.

Uses: Mushrooms can be used in any kind of cooking. They add a delicious taste often called umami. High potency mushrooms can also be purchased in supplement form.

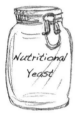

Nutritional Yeast

Benefits: Full of B Vitamins. It's gluten-free, dairy-free and soy-free. Nutritional Yeast is not a yeast, but is a complete protein full of fiber and glutathione.

Uses: A favorite amongst vegans for it's 'cheesy' flavor. Sprinkle on soups, salads and popcorn. Is often added to dips to create depth and a hearty texture.

Oats

Benefits: Oats are full of fiber. They help control blood sugar levels. They are gluten-free unless contaminated during processing.

Uses: Slowly cook and eat as a breakfast cereal, or add to baked goods to increase fiber content. Gently roast and make your own granola bars with them.

Organic Extra Virgin Olive Oil

Benefits: It is full of antioxidants and acts as an anti-inflammatory. Olive oil can help lower cholesterol levels, and prevent heart attacks and strokes.

Uses: Olive oil is a great fat. Don't cook with it, instead drizzle over your food after cooking, and remember to use organic, extra-virgin olive oil.

Onions

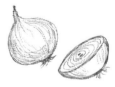

Benefits: Onions are a great source of sulfur compounds. They help reduce blood pressure, lower cholesterol levels, and prevent bone loss in women.

Uses: Onions add a great flavor profile to different dishes. If you find them too pungent, try sweet onion varieties for a gentler flavor.

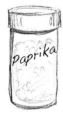

Paprika

Benefits: Paprika has 25% of your daily value of Vitamin A. It acts an anti-inflammatory, boosts circulation, and helps with digestion.

Uses: Paprika adds a tangy flavor to your dishes! Add to homemade tomato sauce. Sprinkle on baked sweet potatoes. Use in chili, soups or stews.

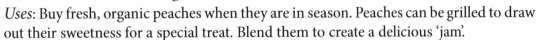

Peaches

Benefits: Peaches have a high amount of potassium, iron, and fiber. They also have 10 different vitamins, including Vitamin C, and act as an antioxidant.

Uses: Buy fresh, organic peaches when they are in season. Peaches can be grilled to draw out their sweetness for a special treat. Blend them to create a delicious 'jam'.

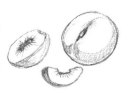

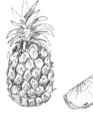

Peas

Benefits: Peas are full of anti-oxidants, fiber, and riboflavin. One cup provides 8.5 grams of protein. They also have anti-inflammatory benefits!

Uses: A great veggie to eat on their own, or can be added to salads, soups and stews. If you like pea-protein, then use fresh or frozen peas instead of the powdered form.

Pecans

Benefits: Pecans help decrease cholesterol levels and provide a lot of vegan protein. They are full of more than 19 vitamins and minerals and have a high amount of Vitamin E.

Uses: Pecans can be crushed and sprinkled into a wide variety of baked goods. Slow cook oats, apples, pecans and cinnamon overnight for a delicious morning porridge.

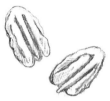

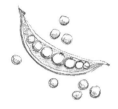

Pineapples

Benefits: They are full of complex B vitamins, Vitamin C, and bromelain (digestive aid). Pineapple acts as an anti-inflammatory and immune booster.

Uses: Pineapples are great fresh and freshly juiced. Pineapple can also enhance different protein-based dishes when baked. Can replace refined sugar while baking.

Pink Himalayan Salt

Benefits: Contains up to 84 minerals, and is known to help balance pH levels. It's minerals are considered colloidal, meaning they are tiny enough for cells to easily absorb.

Uses: Replace traditional sea salt or table salt. Add some to water to enhance electrolytes, reduce cramps and balance blood sugar.

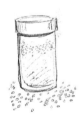

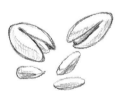

Pistachios

Benefits: Pistachios are a great source of fiber, protein, manganese, and copper. They also contain thiamine, Vitamin B-6, and potassium.

Uses: Use in snack mixes. They also taste delicious in baked goods and homemade ice-cream made with bananas.

Pomegranate

Benefits: Pomegranate also includes many antioxidants. One cup of pomegranate seeds are a good source of potassium, Vitamin C, fiber and protein.

Uses: Pomegranate seeds are delicious by themselves as a snack or when juiced. Add them to salads for beautiful color, flavor and tartness.

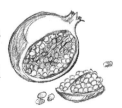

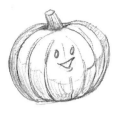

Pumpkin

Benefits: Pumpkin contains high levels of antioxidants, beta-carotene, iron, zinc, Vitamin C and A, and complex B Vitamins.

Uses: Pumpkin is the flavor of fall. It can be made into a variety of baked goods, soups or smoothies. Mashed pumpkin is also a great digestive aid and can relieve constipation.

Pumpkin Seeds

Benefits: Don't throw away those seeds! They provide magnesium and essential fatty acids. They are a natural anti-inflammatory and help lower cholesterol.

Uses: When toasted with your favorite spices, they make a great snack! Eat them raw, or add to snack mixes and granola bars. Sprinkle on salads or add to smoothies.

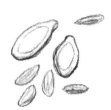

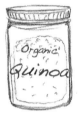

Quinoa

Benefits: A low-glycemic food and complete protein with essential amino acids. It's considered a good source of calcium, iron, phosphorus, and Vitamins B and E.

Uses: Quinoa is a very versatile. It tastes delicious with banana and cinnamon as a morning porridge. Often used in gluten-free baking too.

Raspberries

Benefits: A great source of Vitamin C and dietary fiber. They have a very high ORAC (oxygen radical absorbance capacity) which helps fight off potential cancerous cells.

Uses: These berries taste great fresh and raw. Purchase in bulk when in season and freeze for future use. Add smoothies, juices and baked goods. Excellent on morning porridge.

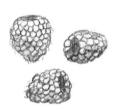

Red Lentils

Benefits: Can help stabilize blood sugar. They are an excellent source of protein and fiber. They are also high in folate, Vitamin A, potassium, magnesium, iron, and anti-oxidants.

Uses: Add to soups or stews. Use to replace flour for gluten-free baking. Create a base for dips and sauces.

Rose Hips

Benefits: Rose hips have more Vitamin C than most citrus fruits and contain important antioxidants.

Uses: Eat fresh and raw, or steep in hot water for a delicious tea.

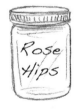

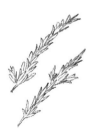

Rosemary

Benefits: Rosemary is rich in Vitamin A and B. It is a good source of dietary fiber. It can help improve memory and fight infections.

Uses: Rosemary is a very well-rounded spice. Add to savory or sweet dishes.

Sesame Seeds (Tahini)

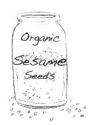

Benefits: These seeds are high in calcium and phytosterol. As an antioxidant, they can help lower cholesterol and reduce inflammation.

Uses: Use Tahini as you would any other nut butter. Add seeds to salads, soups, or your favorite dish. Sprout sesame seeds and sunflower seeds together to make a 'seed cheese'.

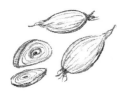

Shallots

Benefits: Shallots are a great source of iron, fiber, folate, and potassium. They have even more antioxidants than onions!

Uses: Shallots can be used in place of onions. They add a nice flavor to other stir fried or sautéed vegetables.

Slippery Elm

Benefits: Slippery elm is a traditional medicinal plant used to treat coughs, stomach troubles, and other health issues.

Uses: Use in cooking porridge, or make your own cough drops.

Spaghetti Squash

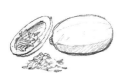

Benefits: One cup of spaghetti squash is an excellent source of Vitamin A, fiber, and magnesium. It's considered an antioxidant and helps reduce inflammation.

Uses: Use spaghetti squash to create a delicious casserole, or eat with your favorite sauce. Use in replacement of regular spaghetti or pasta.

Spinach

Benefits: Spinach is best known for its high amounts of antioxidants, and Vitamin K and A. It also has phytonutrients and antioxidants (helps fight cancerous cells).

Uses: Fresh, organic spinach tastes great as salad greens. Use in omelets and main dishes. You can steam, bake or sauté them.

Spirulina

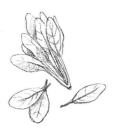

Benefits: Spirulina is a great way to add protein to your meals! It has the same amount of calcium, phosphorus, and magnesium that is found in most milk. It also contains all essential amino acids. It also helps improve the immune system and balances cholesterol.

Uses: Add to smoothies, sprinkle on salads, or add to salad dressing.

Sprouts

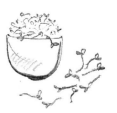

Benefits: These are a concentrated source of vitamins, minerals, amino acids, and enzymes. They're a phenomenal source of chlorophyll.

Uses: Sprouts are a great way to add more nutrition to your salads or fresh made juices. Sprouts are easy to grow and add beauty to your food.

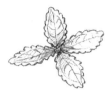

Stevia, Green Leaf or Powder

Benefits: It is a natural alternative to refined or artificial sugars. Be aware that organic green stevia powder is the real thing, and the white powders are highly refined.

Uses: Use as a sugar replacement. Since it's sweeter than refined sugar, experiment with amounts needed to achieve the sweetness you desire.

Strawberries

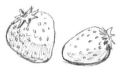

Benefits: Besides being very tasty, strawberries are an excellent source of Vitamin C and manganese. They are full of antioxidants and are anti-inflammatory.

Uses: Strawberries are delicious fresh and freeze well. They taste delicious in smoothies and mixed with banana.

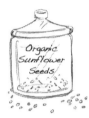

Sunflower Seeds

Benefits: Sunflower seeds provide Vitamin E and complex Vitamin B. They are an excellent source of folic acid and magnesium.

Uses: Sunflower seeds taste great with sliced apples and nut butter. Sprinkle on salads or use in snack mixes. They also make a great seed cheese with sesame seeds.

Sweet Potatoes

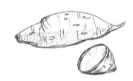

Benefits: These potatoes are high in Vitamins A, C, B5 and B6. They are also a wonderful source of potassium, copper, and manganese. They have anti-inflammatory properties.

Uses: Sweet potatoes are a great starch to add to your meals. They're delicious when added with mashed sweet berries or just a pinch of Celtic Sea Salt.

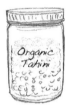

Tahini

Benefits: Like many other foods on this list, it's high in Vitamin E and B. It also contains magnesium, potassium, iron, and calcium.

Uses: It's a great addition to sauces, hummus, and cookies. Throw it on top of cooked vegetables like a sauce!

Tomatoes

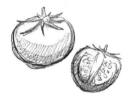

Benefits: Tomatoes are high in Vitamins A and K. They also contain chromium (helps manage blood sugar) and lycopene which combats cancer cells.

Uses: If you can't get fresh tomatoes, buy them in a glass jar only. Make your own tomato sauce, add to salads and savory foods.

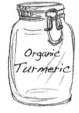

Turmeric

Benefits: This spice is antibacterial, anti-inflammatory, and is an antioxidant. It is great for liver detoxification.

Uses: Use in tonic drinks such as Golden Milk. Mix with a little water and natural sweetener for headache or pain relief. Turmeric is commonly found in curry recipes.

Vanilla Bean Powder

Benefits: Vanilla bean powder has 3 grams of protein and 3 grams of fiber. It's an anti-microbial and antioxidant that helps reduce inflammation.

Uses: This adds a nice flavor to smoothies and baked goods. Vanilla bean powder adds sweetness while cutting down on the need for sugar.

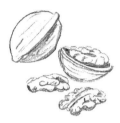

Walnuts

Benefits: Walnuts are high in Vitamin C and Omega-3 fatty acids. They are an excellent vegan source of protein and help improve blood lipids.

Uses: Walnuts make a delicious snack alone or add to salads. Add to baked goods, crumble and use on soups or salads.

Watermelon

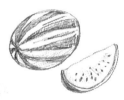

Benefits: Watermelon is high in Vitamin C and potassium. It contains antioxidants which help reduce inflammation, and is also a natural diuretic.

Uses: The best way to enjoy watermelon is to eat it fresh. You can also juice watermelon and it makes for a delicious refreshing summer drink.

Wheatgrass Juice

Benefits: Cleanses kidneys, liver, and the urinary tract. Is an immune-booster and activates the metabolism. Excellent for detoxifying the body and is a complete protein.

Uses: Juice and drink strait. You can also add Wheatgrass juice to your smoothies or fresh juices for an added energy and nutrient boost.

Yacon Syrup

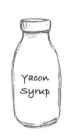

Benefits: Yacon syrup is extracted from the Yacon plant. It's high in fiber and improves digestion, assists blood sugar levels and increases energy.

Uses: Yacon syrup can be used as a sugar alternative and has a creamy caramel taste and texture. Excellent for homemade energy bars and to sweeten warm beverages.

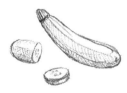

Zucchini

Benefits: Zucchini is high in manganese and potassium. It can help lower blood pressure and is a diabetic friendly food. Full of fiber and nutrients.

Uses: Zucchini can be enjoyed on its own or mixed with other veggies. Try shredding it to create a pasta texture. Bake it, steam it, sauté it or enjoy it raw!

The above is NOT a complete list of nutrient dense foods, nor is it a complete list of their benefits. Be sure to always read ingredients and slowly add in foods you've never eaten before.

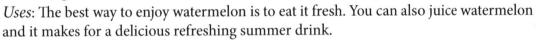

How to Boost Your Energy with Fruit Juices & Smoothies

Do you still believe that a store bought (not freshly made) bottled smoothie or fruit juice is a healthy alternative or energy boost? There is a big difference between a smoothie freshly made with vegetables and fruit, and one made with processed fruit. This goes back to the Magic Trio Combination. Too much simple sugar or fast carbs (pure fruit juice without Fiber, Protein, and Fat to slow it down) gives you a quick rise in blood sugar. But a quick rise means get ready for a quick drop in blood sugar. Excess sugar in the body is stored as fat. As a result, simple sugars and fast carbs increase weight gain because the body has to work harder to process too many simple sugars (why sodas create weight gain instead of weight loss).

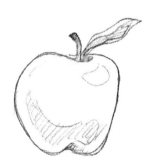

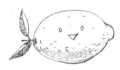

When it comes to fruit juice, consume a small amount but make sure you drink it with a meal or include in a smoothie that also contains Fiber, Protein, and Fat. Remember you want to slow down the digestion of sugars by adding other nutrients. Therefore, a berry smoothie with ground flax seeds assimilates in your body more effectively. As a result, you have **more** energy compared to just drinking a glass of juice.

If you love juice, I recommend switching to fresh squeezed juice (from your own juicer or juice bar) or cold pressed juice. Some health food stores are starting to carry cold pressed juices. Always read ingredients to see what's in them and when they were made. These fresh, cold pressed juices are a wonderful Upgrade from pasteurized bottled juices or juice boxes.

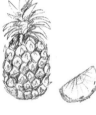

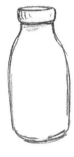

Don't be fooled by the bottles, cartons, or juice boxes that say "Freshly squeezed", "100% juice", or "Not from concentrate". If they sit in a bottle, box, or carton and have an expiration date of more than a few days, then they are pasteurized and altered in order to have a long shelf life. Once pasteurized, they no longer have natural enzymes. When a fruit or vegetable no longer has its natural enzymes, they contain only simple sugar, fructose, and fast carbs. These juices give you a quick burst of energy and then a quick drop of energy. You are better off eating a piece of fruit than drinking enzyme-lacking, and chemically, heat-altered pasteurized drinks.

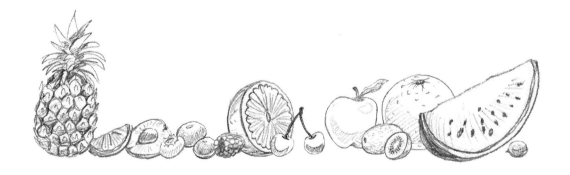

Energizing Drink - Fresh Green Juice

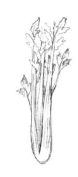

Another great energizing drink is green juice. This is best when made at home or purchased from a juice bar. If you've ever had FRESH green juice (and then let it sit for a while), you will know what REAL juice looks like. It tends to look mostly like water with some stuff hanging out at the bottom until you mix it up again. To keep juice for no more than three days, put some raw honey (not the sugar honey) in the container and store in the refrigerator. After a few days, juice loses many of its nutrients so drink within a short time period. Another way to make a meal out of juice and make it more digestible: take some veggies, add real fruit, then add chia, hemp or ground flax seeds, and blend into a smoothie.

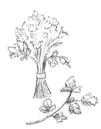

Juicers range in price. If you want to make juice at home and aren't ready to invest in a juicer, use a blender then strain the juice through a nut milk bag. There are many juicers with different functions on the market. Make sure you use a juicer that doesn't heat up the juice. Borrow a juicer to get the hang of it and see which one works for you. Some are easier to clean than others, so keep that in mind when shopping around for a juicer.

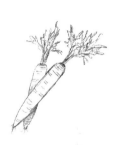

If you like fresh green juice and feel good about it, drink it in the morning or have it for your afternoon snack. Veggies ARE a more efficient energy booster than any caffeine/chocolate/energy drink combined (minus the jitters). Try fresh green juice or chow down on greens (yup, try just greens) the next time you'd normally go for a mid-afternoon, 'fast carb' pick-me-up. You might just be surprised!

While this chapter specifically addresses healing foods, the next chapter gives you helpful shopping, meal planning, and cooking strategies. These tips will set you up for success on your Upgrade journey. Learn how to create your 'I CAN' shopping list, how to shop for organic foods, how to set up your Kitchen Sanctuary (page 189), and the safest cookware to use in your kitchen, etc.

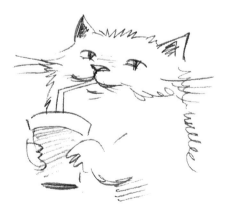

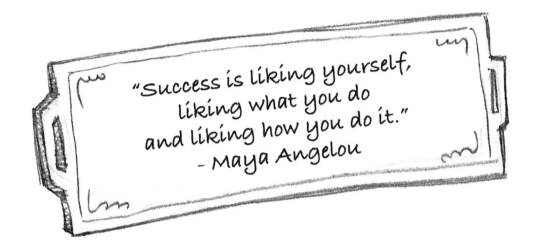

"Success is liking yourself, liking what you do and liking how you do it."
– Maya Angelou

8 SuccesSology

Shopping & Cooking Strategies for Successful Upgrading

This chapter is filled with helpful ideas to motivate you with shopping and cooking strategies and help keep you organized. Remember that organization is your golden ticket to the Upgrade process. Refer to the provided lists and charts to help you along the way. Feel free to use these pages as your personal resource and refer back to them often. Choose just one thing at a time. Start with the I CAN List and continue to slowly Upgrade from there. **Remember that each and every Upgrade IS a SUCCESS!**

I CAN List

The 'I CAN List' is so much better than a "I can't" or a "don't you dare" list. **Remember the purple unicorn exercise** (page 36)? **We think about what we talk about, whether it has I can or I can't OR do or don't in the title**. Instead, talk and think about what you **CAN** have and what you **DO** want!

Use this shopping list or create your own version of the "I CAN List". Keep a copy of it in the kitchen, on the computer, in your car, in your purse/bag, and **any place that inspires you with the foods you CAN enjoy**. I write some of my upgrade items directly on one my canvas shopping bags! Shopping the perimeter of the store is also very helpful. The perimeter of the store will have your fresh fruits,vegetables, and foods that most resemble their natural state. The inner aisles of the store are mostly stocked with processed and refined items (but not always). Remember you can alter this list to suit your specific likes and needs. If there's something on the list you can't stand, cross it out. You can download a version of the "I CAN List" located on the next page from www.Upgradeology.com or www.NicoleWhiteWellness.com.

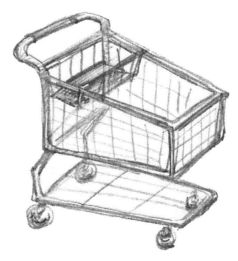

Sweet Veggies
__Carrots
__Beets
__Sweet Potatoes
__Squash
__Bell Peppers
__Pea pods
__Sugar Snap Peas
__Rutabagas
__Jicama

Bulb Veggies
__Asparagus
__Celeriac (celery root)
__Celery
__Chives
__Garlic
__Fennel
__Kohlrabi
__Leeks
__Lemongrass
__Lotus root
__Onions
__Scallions
__Shallots

Greens/Veggies
__Arugula
__Bok Choy
__Broccoli
__Brussels Sprouts
__Cabbage
__Celery
__Collard Greens
__Purslane
__Dandelion
__Kale
__Lettuce
__Mizuna Greens
__Mustard Greens
__Radish
__Spinach
__Swiss Chard
__Turnip
__Watercress

Vegetable/Fruits:
__Tomato
__Avocado
__Bell Pepper
__Eggplant
__Pumpkin
__Squash
__Peppers
__Zucchini

Root Veggies
__Bamboo Shoots
__Burdock
__Carrot
__Daikon
__Ginger
__Horseradish
__Jerusalem Artichoke
__Jicama
__Parsnip
__Rutabaga
__Sweet potato
__Taro
__Turmeric
__Wasabi
__Water Chestnut
__Yacon
__Yams

Vegetables/Flowers
__Artichoke
__Broccoli
__Cauliflower
__Squash Blossoms
__Capers

Sea Vegetables
__Arame
__Dulse
__Hijiki
__Kombu
__Laver
__Nori
__Sea Lettuce
__Wakame
__Kelp

Fruits
__Apples
__Pears
__Apricots
__Peaches
__Figs
__Dates
__Raisins
__Currents
__Cranberries
  (unsweetened)
__Pomegranate
__Melons
__Nectarines
__Papaya
__Pineapple
__Oranges
__Blood Oranges
__Grapes
__Apricots
__Banana
__Cherimoya
__Persimmon
__Plums.

Low Glycemic Fruits
__Berries
__Cherries
__Strawberries
__Raspberries
__Blackberries
__Huckleberries
__Gooseberries
__Lime
__Lemon
__Grapefruit

Legumes
__Azuki
__Black-Eyed Peas
__Chickpeas
__Fava Beans
__Green beans
__Lentils
__Lima Beans
__Mung Beans
__Okra
__Snap Peas
__Kidney Beans

Nuts
__Almond
__Brazil
__Cashew
__Chestnuts
__Filbert
__Hazelnut
__Macadamia
__Pecan
__Pili
__Pine
__Pistachio

Seeds
__Chia
__Flax
__Hemp
__Poppy
__Pumpkin
__Sesame
__Sunflower

Salt:
__Celtic Sea Salt
__Himalayan Salt

Get Organic or Wild Crafted Whenever Possible

Herbs & Spices

__Cinnamon
__Ginger
__Turmeric
__Pepper
__Basil
__Bay Leaf
__Cardamom
__Mustard Seed
__Fenugreek
__Caraway
__Cayenne
__Cilantro

__Chives
__Sage
__Clove
__Coriander Seed
__Cumin
__Dill
__Fennel
__Garlic
__Lavender
__Lemon Verbena
__Licorice Root
__Marjoram
__Mint
__Oregano
__Paprika
__Parsley
__Peppermint
__Rosemary
__Saffron
__Sage
__Star Anise
__Tarragon
__Thyme
__Vanilla
__Wasabi
__Savory

Upgraded Sweeteners

__Organic Black Strap Molasses
__Organic Date Sugar
__Organic Local Raw Honey
__Organic Maple Syrup
__Organic Coconut Sugar
__Organic Coconut Palm Sugar
__Organic Dates
__Organic Green Stevia Powder
__Yacon Syrup
__Lacuma

Oil / Nourishing Fats

__Organic Extra Virgin Olive Oil,
__Organic Extra Virgin Coconut OIL
__Organic Pasture Raised UNSALTED Butter (add your own sea salt)
__Organic Ghee, Organic Pasture, Raised Lard (if you are going to cook using high heat such as frying)
__Avocado (also Chia Seeds and Flax Seeds for Fat)

Condiments

__Organic Apple Cider Vinegar (use in place of white vinegar)
__Nutritional Yeast (can be used in place of cheese)
__Organic Wheat Free Tamari (use instead of soy sauce)
__Coconut Secret Raw Coconut Aminos (use instead of soy sauce)
__Miso: South River Miso (variety of flavors), Miso Masters Miso Soup

Animal Products

Organic, Pasture Raised, Hormone Free, Antibiotic Free, Free Range, NON-GMO Feed animal products:
__Eggs
__Meats
__Poultry
__Wild Caught Fish

Dairy

Organic, Grass Fed, Hormone & Anti-biotic FREE
__Unsweetened/Plain Yogurt
__Cheese
__Milk

Sheep or Goat

__Plain Yogurt
__Raw Cheese
__RAW Milk

Get Organic Whenever Possible

Always Read Ingredients

Notes from the I CAN List

Canned: If you buy canned products, be sure to read the ingredients and make sure they are BPA-free cans (it's best if they are organic). If canned items contain salt, rinse with filtered water before using (this helps reduce table salt content). **Fresh & Organic is #1**, Next is organic frozen, Last is organic canned.

RAW or Roasted and UN-salted Nuts

Upgrade to organic, raw, and then sprouted, see sprouting information below. **Note:** Peanuts are actually a legume, I recommend using Almond/Almond Butter, Sunflower Seeds, or Seed Butters instead.

How to Grow Your Own Sprouts

Growing your own sprouts is very easy, inexpensive and extremely nutritious. At first it may *seem* complicated, but after you do it once, you'll see that it's quite easy. Because it is a detailed oriented process I'd like to guide you over to www.sproutpeople.org for all of your sprouting instructions and needs! I've listed the bare bones of sprouting here:

1. Use one part seed to at least 3 parts water.
2. Soak seeds (time depends on seed/bean) in a wide-mouth jar.
3. Drain the soaking water.
4. Rinse the bean/seed 2-3 times a day.
5. Watch your sprouts grow, then eat and enjoy!

Seeds	Soak Time	Days to Sprout
* 2 TBSP red clover	6 hours	5-6 days
* 1/4 cup radish or mustard	6 hours	5-6 days
* 1/2 cup lentils or fenugreek	8 hours	3 days
* 1/2 cup mung beans	8 hours	3-5 days
* 1 cup aduki, garbanzo	12 hours	3-5 days
* 2 cups sunflower seeds	12 hours	2 days

How to Prepare Frozen Meals

Allow frozen meals to thaw before you heat them in the oven. Use glass or ceramic containers – never use metal or plastic. Heating in the oven is preferable. If you are limited and can only use a microwave, let the item thaw out completely and only heat for less than one minute. I never use a microwave, but I understand that it's the only option people have if they work in an office. Ask if your office will provide a toaster oven. These are much, much better, and toaster ovens are very inexpensive.

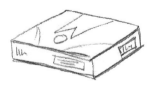

If you tend to eat a lot of frozen meals at home, buy the best organic brand and invest in a toaster oven at home (if you don't want to use your oven). Even better, use a slow cooker. Yes, certain frozen entrées and soups can be put into a slow cooker. You will need to add some water but it works. Bring your slow cooker to work, especially if you have your own office.

Cooking Hints

✳ **Choose a texture that you like as the base:**
i.e. kidney beans, brown rice, grass fed organic beef, etc.

✳ **Add vegetables:**
Pile in the vegetables. Prepare them according to your preference i.e. steam, sauté, bake, etc.

✳ **Add sauce:**
Make sure that the sauce tastes really great because this ties the dish together.

✳ **Use Celtic Sea Salt or Himalayan Salt to bring out the natural flavors of your food.**

✳ **Slow cooking foods also bring out the flavor and delicious texture in foods.** Use a slow cooker/crock pot for one pot meals or slowly cook on the stove-top.

✳ **Add organic, clean ingredient condiments to make your food taste the way you like it.**

Not only will you reap the health benefits by upgrading to quality, nourishing organic foods (see Organics, page 56), but organics are more affordable than you think. Thankfully, more and more people are becoming aware and supporting organics. The more people that support smaller, organic farms, the more their crops are used and consumed. As a result, they are encouraged to continue farming the land. I quoted it before but it's worth repeating again: *You can pay the farmer, or you can pay the Doctor!*

The Why Upgrade List...

Many people find it helpful to have a list of foods that they used to eat, love and crave. See Foods below with known symptoms listed next to them.

It's helpful to keep these charts handy, and makes it easier for you to reference the I CAN LIST (page 182). It also acts as a reminder of foods that are healing and helpful, so you don't have to dwell on the foods you are upgrading from.

Food Item	Side Effects - Side Effects - Side Effects
Refined Sugar	Foggy vision, irritability, restlessness, moodiness, Candida, never ending cravings, overeating, and inability to see the benefit of eating healthy foods
Wheat	Bloating, brain fog, turns to sugar with similar effects in body, trouble getting up in the morning
Coffee	Jitters, paranoia, go too long without eating then overeat in the evening, metallic feeling in the mouth, insomnia, low energy
Fast Food	Brain fog, bloating, excessive weight gain, joint pain, blurry vision, headaches, allergies, bad body odor
Dairy	Bloating, headache, eczema, allergies, flatulence, craving for more
Diet Soda	Severe wrist pains, false carpal tunnel, jitters, inflammation and major joint pain, headaches, moodiness/irritability, insomnia, hormonal issues and the farts.

Old	Upgraded
Refined Sugar	Organic Coconut Sugar or Raw Honey
Wheat	Gluten Free Grains, Quinoa, Brown Rice, Amaranth
Coffee	Green tea, Chicory Root, Coconut water, Cacao/Coconut Sugar/Coconut Butter
Fast Food	Pre-planned, slow cooked meals or shop at the natural market to see what choices they have. Call a quality restaurant for a 'to-go' order.
Dairy	Organic Grass Fed Dairy, Sheep, Goat, Nut/Seed/Coconut milks/butters
Diet Soda	Kombucha, bubbly water with blueberries in it

Helpful Organic Shopping Tips

Organization is the key to eating organic on a budget!

Sale/Coupons

If you are a coupon person or love to shop at natural food markets, plan out your meals for the week based on coupons or store items that are on sale.

Budget

Track how much you spend on food and drink for one week. That includes every coffee shop, vending machine, take-out, grocery store, restaurant, etc. Tally up how much you spend on everything! When you add up your food and drink purchases for the week, you'll realize it's usually cheaper to buy organics and make your own meals, snacks, and drinks and take them with you. If money is your biggest worry with organics, then I challenge you to see where you spend your food, drink, and medication money. With some careful planning, you can eat organic, feel better, and will likely spend less money than you currently spend on foods and drinks.

Going Out - Your Third Place

Do you love the coffee shop where everyone knows your name and your drink? Do you enjoy eating out? Do you like to meet friends for a meal or drink at your favorite place? I urge you to think about why you love those places. For many of my clients, that morning coffee shop is their few moments of comfort before diving into their workday. It's that place where you enjoy spending time. Sometimes referred to as the "Third Place" (First being home and second being work). There is usually a good feeling about this "Third Place" which encourages you to return often.

How can you create this same third place experience? Choose any of the tips below that appeal to you.

* Turn your house into your favorite restaurant by mimicking the recipes of your favorite foods at home.

* Budget special occasions and create a fun restaurant night at your house…"play" when the world meets your eye like a big pizza pie, that's amore!

* Buy organic tea, keep it with you, and ask for hot water at tea or coffee houses. Save moolah and give the barista a buck tip. It's still cheaper and you have your third place.

* Make your own granola bars and carry goodie snacks with you. See **Gotta Go Bag** (page 118) for more ideas.

* If you can't afford the fresh organics, look for frozen alternatives.

* Make homemade goodies and freeze the extras so you can pull out of the freezer or bake when you want them.

* When your favorite fruits or vegetables are on sale, buy them in bulk quantity and freeze them yourself (i.e. berries freeze well)!

How to Get Organized

Choose any of these items that appeal to you. These aren't listed in any particular order, and you don't have to incorporate all of them. Begin with just one.

* Cook once and eat multiple times. When cooking, make enough for two or three nights. If you really love the dish, freeze some for another time (especially if you don't like eating the same meal a few days in a row).

* Always choose the highest quality animal and dairy products. As a kid, I'd save the best tasting item on my plate for last. I'd eat a little throughout the meal but would make sure that the last bite was delicious. When you include meat or dairy in your meals, make them a sprinkle of your food. Ever notice how specialty foods always taste better when there are less of them? Organic beans and whole grains are inexpensive, simple to cook, and very filling.

* Check to see if any of your 'staples' are on sale and stock up on these items.

* Try to buy locally whenever you can! If you don't know what is available in your community check out localharvest.org and get to know your farmers. Better yet, visit your local Farmer's Market. Some Farmers Markets are Certified Organic while others are conventional. Some farmers are certified organic, and others don't use spray and are organic without the expensive certifications.

* Another way to save money is to go to the Farmer's Market just before they close. Most farmers prefer to sell leftovers at a lower price rather than load and unload their products again.

* Ask the folks at the grocery store what they do with the produce that isn't good enough to display anymore. These items are usually sold at a major discount, and you can often get them super cheap or even free. Remember that slightly wilted or bruised Organic produce is better than the 'prettiest' looking conventional item. (Refer to Organics on page 56 for more tips).

* Join your local CSA (Community Supported Agriculture) or join the United Buying Club (unitedbuyingclubs.com) for delicious fresh food.

* If you have some time and land, consider starting your own little garden with NON-GMO seeds. Again, the Internet has endless information on how to start small with a pesticide-free garden. Start with a small jar of sprouts then add an herb garden in the window or perhaps a few pots on the front porch. Compost any food waste. Composting returns nutrients back to your soil instead of dumping them into landfills. Composting is not always accessible for people, but you can seek out people who want your compost.

* If you love eggs and have the room, consider getting chickens. You can feed chickens leftover produce scraps. In return, they will give you eggs. If you have never had pasture raised eggs, compare them sometime to what you get in the store and be prepared to be wow'd! The yolks in regular eggs will be pale, while the yolks in pasture raised eggs will be golden yellow/orange.

* Consider canning or preserving your own food. There is so much FREE information on the internet on how to can, ferment, and preserve foods you grow or purchase in bulk. You also know what's in it when you can or ferment food yourself. See Sauerkraut recipe in Probiotic Foods (Chapter 5, page 124).

* Traveling and eating organic can be tricky! One of my favorite tips is to add Chia Seeds to a bottle of water when traveling. This helps you stay hydrated on the plane. If you are careful to follow TSA guidelines, you can bring many of your favorite foods with you in a small cooler. Some other great travel tips can be found on my website, www.Upgradeology.com or www.NicoleWhiteWellness.com

* Bring filtered water with you wherever you go, and always carry snacks with you! See Snacks (page 114) and Gotta Go Bag (page 118) for more ideas.

* The pre-washed and fancy packaged fruits and veggies are always more expensive. These are okay options once in a while. However, if money is an issue it's far less expensive to wash, cut, and package your own produce.

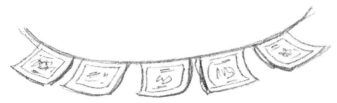

Kitchen Sanctuary

It's important that you set up your home to be an Upgraded food environment. When I still ate pastries, I'd actually go to the grocery store every night and buy one. Yes, it would have been much cheaper to buy the four pack; however, if I had the four pack at home at least 3 or 4 would be gone by the evening. And if they were still there in the morning, then they would be my breakfast too. I've known for a long time that the things I eat at night when I'm not feeling well are not things that should linger around in the morning.

This is why your kitchen sanctuary is so important. For me, it's important that I only bring home nourishing foods. I have a deal with myself. If I want something junky – that's fine but it doesn't come home with me. That way, every morning my only options are Upgraded ones. This is a challenge for many people, especially for my clients, because they live with other people who are not on board with Upgraded eating habits.

Here are some tips to set up your kitchen:

* Have your own cabinet, or at least a shelf, that is for your food only.
* Have your own space in the refrigerator or freezer that is only for YOU!

I had a client come back with: "well, then they eat my food!" This is actually a good thing! If family members or roommates are going to eat your Upgraded foods, then buy more nourishing REAL foods and less of the fake, chemically-processed ones! The less that stuff is in your kitchen, the better!

This does take some time and careful planning. Most importantly, communicate with the people you live with or who share your food storage. However, this is one of the most important things you can do to ensure success. If your only options for breakfast are Upgraded ones that taste delicious to you, then you are more likely to begin your day with success. If you are constantly surrounded by foods that bring you down and start your day on a sugar or frankenfood spike, then it's less likely you will stick to Upgrades for the rest of the day.

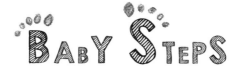

What, if any, are your obstacles at home for having a Kitchen Sanctuary or an Upgraded Kitchen?

What is one little thing you can do to ensure that you have Upgraded breakfast options in your home? Upgraded food that you love, enjoy, and will eat?

Take one little step towards Kitchen Sanctuary. Have your own cabinet or shelf. Ask others to hide their junk food. Get a mini-fridge for yourself, and a padlock that someone else has the combo to for the 'junk food' in the house. Sometimes you have to go to extreme measures.

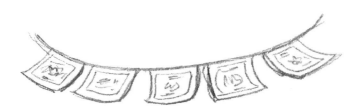

Our homes have to be our **sanctuary**. If junk foods call out your name in the middle of the night and you have easy access to them, then it's easy to give into temptation. If you have trouble figuring out your food situation at home: begin to write down all of your obstacles. Then address them, one by one, to see what your options are. You can do this! Writing them out will help you 100 times MORE than just letting the thoughts swirl around and around in your head.

Food Prep Guide

* Shop local and organic when you can.

* Plan ahead! Make a meal plan and a shopping list.

* Go to the store on a full belly and always have a list with you.

* If produce that you like is on sale then buy it.

* If it's boxed, packaged, new and/or on sale, first look at the ingredients. If they are super clean foods, then go for it. If they have iffy ingredients, then put them back on the shelf. Barter with yourself that you will find yourself a better treat. Keep upgraded 'treats' at the top of your list to refer back to when sales and advertising temptations try to take hold.

* Stick to your 'I Can List' (page 182) as much as you can, especially if snack foods begin to sneak into your cart when you are not looking!

* If you are super busy and/or don't like to cook and shop, do your food prep in one day. At first it will take some time, but you will get into a rhythm and it will get you into the groove.

* Make it a fun adventure! Play music, or an inspirational audio in the car that you love to put you in the mood before you buy nourishing foods.

* While in the kitchen, play a great audio book or inspiring music. This helps put you in a good mood and keeps you motivated.

* Clean the kitchen and fridge *before* going to the grocery store. Set up your kitchen to wash and store produce as soon as you get home. Nothing is worse than finding rotted organic veggies in the back of the fridge (I know this from experience).

Produce Prep Tips

After shopping, wash and separate your produce into bags or containers (or have one large container for various produce) for each day of the week. 'Debbie Meyer' bags are a great way to preserve produce. I have a friend who goes to the market once a week on Sundays. When she gets home, she washes and sorts everything. She looks at her menu for the week and then sorts and bags up the ingredients she will need for each day's meal. She even puts little baggies of spices inside the bags. Each morning, she then takes out the contents and puts them in a slow cooker. When she gets home at night, she has an amazing slow cooked meal. Brilliance!

This is a helpful idea for folks who love organization and don't want to waste a morsel of food. I personally tend to wing it, but I also enjoy cooking on a daily basis. At the beginning, I highly recommend planning ahead. Do whatever works to get you motivated in the kitchen. Go for it! Otherwise, clean produce as you bring it home and store it in containers so you have easy access.

Cook for the week, separate and freeze the dishes, then warm up in the oven or stove-top on the day you plan to eat them. It's a good idea to label with dates and possible ingredients, just in case you find it two months from now (embarrassingly speaking from experience here).

Notes on Parasites

To avoid parasites and other undesirables on your raw fruits and vegetables, clean all fruits and veggies well. The best way to do this is get a large bowl or fill a clean sink and plug with water. Add 1/4 TBSP of Food Grade Hydrogen Peroxide **per** gallon of water. Let the fruits and veggies soak in this mixture of water and hydrogen peroxide for at least 15-20 minutes. They are then good to go. I prefer to soak mine in filtered water with hydrogen peroxide. Look for 'Food Grade Hydrogen Peroxide' online or in health food stores. This is an excellent option for thoroughly cleaning raw fruits and vegetables. As often as I can, when I get home from produce shopping, I will wash the produce immediately. This saves me time when I am ready to prepare food.

Cookware

If you make an effort to Upgrade the foods you eat, think about upgrading HOW you cook. Your kitchen and kitchen tools are part of the improved food rituals you are cultivating. You don't have to make these changes all at once, but if you invest in quality kitchen tools it will save you in the long run.

When selecting pots and pans, keep these tips in mind. Over time, due to scratches, the material from your cookware will end up in your food. If your pans are made of aluminum or have a teflon coating, this is dangerous. Teflon can leach into food, and at high temperatures it's extremely toxic. The main chemical in teflon (non-stick) cookware, PFOA (Perfluorooctanoic acid), has been linked to cancer and other serious diseases. Once this chemical is in your system it's very difficult to detox it out. According to Dr. Mercola, consistent exposure to aluminum has been linked to possible neurological issues such as dementia, autism, and possibly Parkinson's disease.

Stainless steel and/or cast iron are great alternatives. Cast iron is heavy but very affordable. I recommend buying a brand made in the USA and follow instructions on how to re-season. They use the cheapest oils to pre-season them, and you don't want to cook in that. A quality stainless steel is much lighter than cast iron and cooks well. If you can afford it, look into the latest technology of ceramic cookware as well. It's made with non-toxic materials and can withstand high heat without cracking or leaching into your food. Remember the old glass cookware? If you can find it, they are wonderful as well.

I recommend glass or non-toxic ceramic (lead-free glazes) bake-ware for cooking and reheating food. Glass will have no flavor transfer, can easily be stored in the refrigerator, and last for years.

When it comes to appliances in the kitchen, keep them fairly simple.

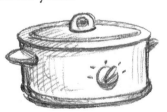

* A high speed blender works wonders.
* A food processor is helpful if you like to bake.
* A slow cooker is essential if you want easy and nourishing foods.
* A hand-held (stainless steel) blender (also called an immersion blender) is helpful for creating hot, pureed foods. The hand held part may be plastic, but make sure that the shaft and blade are stainless steel.
* I don't ever recommend using plastic when using any kind of heat.

You might notice your go-to appliance is missing from this list—the microwave. I know you may think you can't live without your microwave, but I assure you that you can and you will feel better. When you microwave items, it changes the chemical make-up of your food or drink. There is such a thing as microwave sickness too. As with everything, do your own research on anything that doesn't resonate with you.

I understand that sometimes, due to time or being away from your kitchen, using the microwave seems necessary. IF it is your only option for cooking or heating food, I urge you to ONLY use the microwave for very short amounts of time. It's do-able. It's been over 15 years since I've used a microwave. When you decide it's time to go microwave-free, check to make sure the places where you dine are also microwave-free.

A blender or food processor will assist you in making sauces and condiments with confidence and ease. I had a small bullet blender for many years and recently upgraded to a high speed blender. Blendtec and Vitamix are two high speed blender companies that have extremely durable products. Vitamix also has re-furbished units for half the price of a brand new one. These are often used for in-store demonstrations. They are perfectly clean when you get them. They are as good as new AND half the price.

The beauty of a good blender is that all you have to do is throw in the ingredients, hit that button and ta-da! A delicious, nutritious addition to your meal! The same goes for a crockpot (slow cooker). While the Crockpot takes a long time to cook your food, with proper planning the night before or in the morning, you return home to a hot, Upgraded meal for dinner. If you love oatmeal, then you will love waking up to warm, slow cooked oats in the morning. (See page 134 'Morning Apple Pie' recipe)

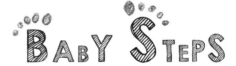

Use what you have on hand right now and begin to make a few simple recipes and Upgrades. There are many recipes that can be created without fancy cookware. You can also check out your local health food store to see what pre-made foods they carry.

If you don't already have the cookware mentioned, slowly Upgrade your kitchen. What's the most important tool for you? After you make your decision, save for it, look for coupons, research online, and then buy it.

Create a schedule for when you plan to make these Upgrades and budget accordingly. If you don't like to cook, see if there is someone who will cook for you or if you can afford it, hire someone to cook for you or teach you how to cook. Share this book with anyone you work with that prepares food for you or with you.

Food Plan

By creating a food plan ahead of time, you will have wide variety of options at your fingertips. If you are not prepared, you will eat what is on hand or unhealthy, processed foods advertised in the supermarket. Rebel against the advertising and BE PREPARED!

When it comes to planning your food options, don't worry about portions. Just focus on eating a quality breakfast so that you start the day SATISFIED! See Breakfast section on page 158 for tips. Eat the quantity that feels good and satisfies you. Remember the most important part of the Upgrade process: first, you must enjoy the taste of your food and be satisfied with the quantity. Otherwise, it's a Diet

Diet = DIE with a capital T for Torture!

*Remember to include The Magic Trio Combination of Fiber, Protein. and Fat (page 101) with every meal and snack for blood sugar stabilization and increased energy.

FOOD PLAN SAMPLE
Write down at least 7-10 different options for Breakfast, Lunch, Dinner and Snacks options that appeal to you.

Breakfast Options:

Lunch Options:

Dinner Options:

Snack Options:

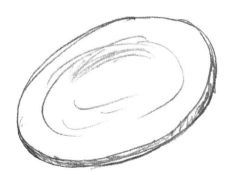

Breakfast Options

Examples:

Omelet
Fiber: Big handful of fresh organic Spinach and Arugula
Protein: 3 Organic Pastured raised eggs
Fat/Sauce: Organic Ghee or Coconut Oil (to cook the omelet)
Spices: Celtic Sea Salt and Organic Pepper, fresh chopped Basil or Parsley on top

Yogurt
Protein: Organic Full Fat Sheep Yogurt or Coconut Yogurt
Fat/Sauce: Organic Ground Flax Seeds
Spices: Organic Ceylon Cinnamon

Now try some from the foods you enjoy!

Fiber:

Protein:

Fat/Sauce:

Spice:

Fiber:

Protein:

Fat/Sauce:

Spice:

Fiber:

Protein:

Fat/Sauce:

Spice:

Lunch & Dinner Options

Examples:

F i b e r : Steamed Carrots, Broccoli, Cauliflower, and Collard Greens and grilled Onions
(Vegetables are also protein)

Protein: 1/4 lb. Organic Pasture-Raised Meat or Poultry

Fat/Sauce: Cumin Avocado Dressing (see Recipe below)

Spices: Celtic Sea Salt or Herbs (sprinkled on top)

Cumin Avocado Dressing

* 1 tsp ground cumin seeds
* 3 TBSP organic lime juice (freshly squeezed)
* 3 TBSP organic extra virgin olive oil
* 1 organic avocado
* 1/2 tsp organic Dijon mustard
* 1 organic garlic clove, minced
* 1/4 cup purified water
* 1/2 tsp Celtic Sea Salt
* Black pepper to taste

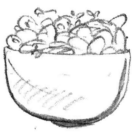

Directions:

1. Blend all ingredients together (except black pepper) until smooth.
2. Add more water until desired consistency. Add pinch of black pepper to taste.

F i b e r : Large bowl of mixed greens, shredded carrots, celery, and cucumber

Protein: Organic black beans and Quinoa

Fat/Sauce: Tahini Dressing (below)

Spices: Celtic Sea Salt and fresh basil

Tahini Dressing

* 1 cup organic tahini
* 1/2 cup organic lemon juice (fresh squeezed)
* 1 organic garlic clove
* ½ cup purified water
* Celtic Sea Salt and organic pepper to taste

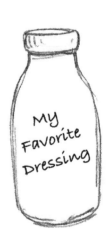

My Favorite Dressing

Directions:

1. Blend all ingredients (except water) together in a bowl or blender.
2. Add water 1 TBSP at a time until desired consistency.
   I like mine thick, while others like their dressing thinner.

Now try some Lunch & Dinner options from the foods you enjoy!

Fiber:

Protein:

Fat/Sauce:

Spice:

Fiber:

Protein:

Fat/Sauce:

Spice:

Fiber:

Protein:

Fat/Sauce:

Spice:

Fiber:

Protein:

Fat/Sauce:

Spice:

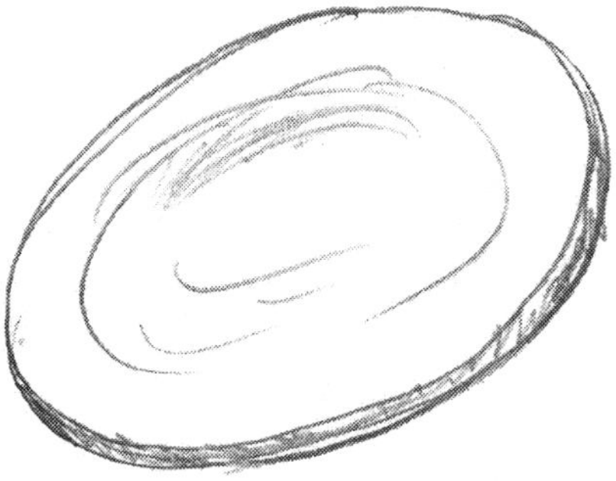

Snack OPTIONS

Examples:

Snack 1:
Fiber/Protein/Fat: Avocado
Spice: Celtic Sea Salt

Snack 2:
Fiber/Protein/Fat: Chia Seeds
Spice: Cinnamon
16 oz water

Snack 3:
Fiber: Sliced carrots
Protein: Hummus
Fat/Sauce: Olive Oil in Hummus
Spice: Celtic Sea Salt

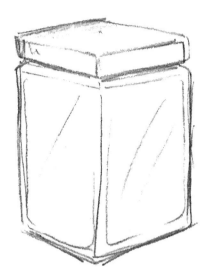

Snack 4:
Fiber: Apple
Protein: Unsalted Nut Butter
Fat/Sauce: Unsalted Nut Butter
Spice: Cinnamon, Celtic Sea Salt

Now try some Lunch & Dinner options from the foods you enjoy!

Fiber:

Protein:

Fat/Sauce:

Spice:

Fiber:

Protein:

Fat/Sauce:

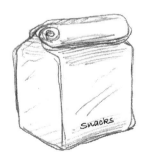

Spice:

Keep It Simple!

* **Upgrade the foods you love!**

* **Create a simple breakfast that satisfies you and stick with it.**

* **Then create simple snacks that you enjoy and keep them with you.**

* **The simpler and more consistent you keep your food, the easier it is to prepare it and stick with it.**

* **Baby Steps, Baby Steps, Baby Steps!**

In Chapter 8 we discussed:

* Shopping and cooking strategies for successful Upgrading
* Your I CAN List and how it's essential
* The Upgraded way to prepare frozen meals
* Cooking tips and tricks
* Why Upgrading is important
* Helpful shopping tips
* What to do when going out, finding your Third Place
* Kitchen Sanctuary
* Food prep guide
* Upgrade your cookware
* Importance of a Food Plan

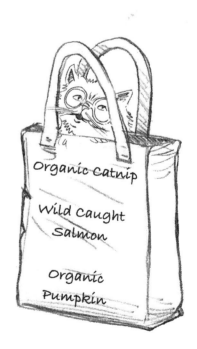

The shopping, cooking and food planning tools detailed above will assist you in your Upgrade success. Remember, you don't need to do them ALL at once. Take just one baby step at a time! During the Upgrade process, it's important to supplement with movement/exercise (appropriate to your body type and lifestyle), meditation, and nourishing ways to reduce stress in your life, etc. The suggestions offered in Chapter 9 are NOT a "one-size-fits-all" approach to your well-being. Pick and choose what works best for your personal lifestyle. Make sure you choose activities that feed your passions and make you feel energized!

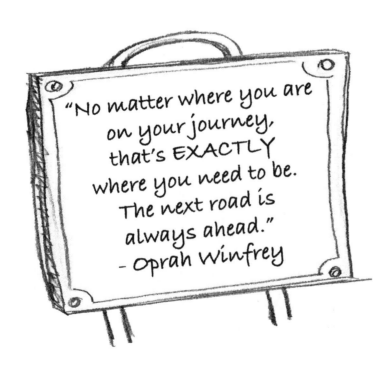

"No matter where you are on your journey, that's EXACTLY where you need to be. The next road is always ahead."
- Oprah Winfrey

9 WELLNESSOLOGY

Tips For Whole Body Wellness

You ARE That Magic Pill!

Your ability to investigate symptoms from the root is that magic pill that you've been looking for all your life. We are constantly bombarded with the new diets, pills, and potions that claim to decrease cravings, release the weight, and make us healthy and happy. Sadly, there are also surgeries and various procedures that promise us the same thing. If these really worked, we'd all be in perfect health. The answer to many of our health and weight issues is a simple one, but not always easy or as convenient as a pill.

I heard a radio talk show host speak about this very topic. She followed a person who was always selling the next wonder drug, super supplement, magic food, 'make you thin' sweetener, exploring the next 'perfect diet', etc. It was refreshing to hear her talk about all the different things she bought into and how NONE of them worked. Do you often think maybe I just didn't stick with it or take enough of it? Or "I wonder why it didn't work for me, what did I do wrong"? But she spoke the truth – all these magic potions are just 'snake oil'. There is no magic pill, because the symptoms you experience are caused by a deeper issue. When you get to the root of the problem and work on it from the inside out, instead of trying to mask it, that's when clarity and healing begin. The process does take patience, planning, experimentation and investigation. This chapter will show you how to discover what baby steps to take, and how to slowly or quickly transition.

I believe that everything happens for a reason. All your symptoms happen for a reason, and the way you resolve your health issues also happen for a reason. I believe that we are healthier than we give ourselves credit for. Begin to notice all the things you do effortlessly such as breathing, walking, talking, moving, etc.

The previous chapters show you how to alter habits and embrace new rituals by Upgrading from fake, processed foods to REAL nourishing foods, but don't forget that you need to nurture your WHOLE body (emotionally, physically and spiritually). This last chapter shows you nourishing, healing Upgrades and tips that support you on your journey…beyond just food and eating habits.

Restful Sleep Rituals

There was a guy who I knew that had a dangerous case of sleep apnea. A health expert in town encouraged him to transition to a nourishing way of eating. With the help of people around him, they cleaned out his kitchen, brought him organic foods and produce, invited him over for meals, and really helped him with his transformation. Within four days of eliminating processed and toxic foods, and eating mostly plant based foods, his sleep apnea disappeared!

9 - Wellnessology

Before electricity, most people lived according to the circadian rhythm (the rise and set of the sun). This is especially difficult for many of us artsy types, as we love the quiet beauty of the evening. Sometimes you have to just flow with a project. I know that I am dedicated to my sleep schedule, but if I haven't been able to write or draw all day and then the *pow of flow* enters my room at 10 pm, I cannot ignore it. I do my best to rise at 6 am and get to sleep by 10 pm, but that's not always the case. Without attempting this schedule, I can be up until 3-4 am. which actually shortens my day and I don't feel well if I sleep until noon. I feel my best on the days I wake up at dawn and am asleep by 10 pm.

Upgrading your sleep takes time and planning. Begin by choosing just one of the items below to guide you on your way towards more restful sleep.

Comfort is key to restful sleep. First, Upgrade your sheets and pajamas to cotton (organic cotton if possible). Cotton or a natural fiber allows airflow and INCREASES circulation. Cotton breathes more than synthetic materials. The next time you are in the market for a new bed, buy an organic cotton mattress or mattress topper.

Add movement into your day. Studies have repeatedly shown that people who exercise are able to fall asleep easier, and sleep more soundly. Even a short, relaxing walk after dinner can assist in better quality sleep. See Movement section on page 216.

How to Prepare for Sleep (2-3 hours before bed) zzZ Z

Begin by choosing one of the following:

* Take Magnesium – A natural relaxation mineral. Most people are extremely magnesium deficient. You can find magnesium in the following foods:
  * Seaweeds: Kelp and Dulse
  * Algae: Spirulina
  * Nuts: Almonds, Cashews, Brazil Nuts, Filberts, Pecans, Walnuts, Sunflower Seeds
  * Produce: Collard Greens, Parsley, Dandelion Greens, Avocados, Garlic, Dates, Figs
  * Whole Grains: Buckwheat, Brown Rice, Millet (Glutenous grains: Rye, Barley)
  * Red Lentils

* Epsom salt baths are high in magnesium. If these don't work, consider a high quality pure magnesium powder or supplement.

* Turn off all electronics 1-2 hours before bed. Electronics stimulate you! See if you can remove yourself from technology at night so you can slowly unwind for peaceful sleep. Lower the lights, take a bath, read a book (not an e-reader), work on a craft, write about your day, listen to soft music, or talk with a friend or family member.

* How to deal with that second wind. When it happens, begin to notice the signs and allow yourself to slow down. Turn off electronics when you reach that first slowdown in the evening.

  For example: You are exhausted at 8pm, but get that second wind at 9pm. Once your second wind comes around you then stay up till 11, midnight or later.

Consider that low point at 8 pm as your sign to start relaxing. You may think that watching TV is relaxing but really it's very stimulating, especially TV with commercials. Commercials are louder with flashing and flickering visuals which are intentional to capture your attention and keep you engaged. Begin to relax by turning off all electronics at that 8pm time. Read a book (real book, not an electronic gadget), engage in a hobby, journal or talk with a loved one.

* Drink Golden Milk at night (see recipe in page 236). You may be delightfully surprised at the results. This is my go-to drink for aches, pains, menstrual issues, fatigue, or when I feel cold. Remember you can play around with the recipe and make it to your liking!

* Quit any and all stimulants by 11 am. If you have trouble sleeping, see if you can have that morning caffeine extra early. Slowly wean yourself to just one cup early in the morning, and leave at least 14 hours for your system to detox from caffeine. If you know it's time to Upgrade those stimulants, see Coffee Upgrades (page 142). If you must have caffeine, have it before 11 am. If you get the afternoon slumps, figure out when those happen and begin to drink water and eat an Upgraded snack BEFORE your slump happens. It will take some time for you to adjust but it works more effectively than stimulants. This includes caffinated tea, chocolate, soft drinks, or smoking cigarettes. Caffeine is a stimulant and if you have any sleep issues, caffeine just might be the root of the problem.

* Let your bedroom be your bedroom, not a TV room, computer room, etc. This is tough for some people. A client lives in a studio so I suggested that she turn everything off at night. Turn off the computer, modem, and printer, and unplug anything that isn't necessary to have on. I suggested keeping the room dark at night and to make sure no computer fans or electronics were running. Some people benefit from playing soothing music to help them relax before bed.

* A white noise machine, sleep mask, earplugs, or sleep enhancing background music will help your brain slowly begin to relax. Search the internet for soundtracks that are specifically designed to help with sleep and relaxation.

* Take a warm bath with Epsom salts (magnesium) and lavender to relax after a long day. Epsom salt baths are an effective way to increase magnesium in the body and promote restfulness. Before bed, place a hot pad on your belly. Rub coconut oil or sesame seed oil and essential oil of lavender on your feet. Lavender oil is calming and encourages sleep.

* Write it down, get it out. Write down all things swirling around in your mind. Sometimes it's our thoughts and worries that keep us awake at night. By writing them down, you get these thoughts out of your system which helps your brain relax and let go. If you know your mind races at night, then write down all of your thoughts and worries before bed. Write out some solutions and when you feel complete and more relaxed, then set them aside and go to sleep.

* If you can't figure out why you still can't sleep, review your day and see if you had any stimulants such as chocolate, tea, coffee or an 'energy drink' that may keep you from the zzzz's. If I have any green tea or cacao after 11 am, it usually disrupts my sleep. If you usually have stimulants after 11 am, write down your plan for the next day. Incorporate energy foods and drinks (without caffeine) to help you with energy which assists with better sleep.

* Assess your alcohol use. When first drinking alcohol, it can make you feel relaxed and sleepy, but it actually elevates your temperature and interferes with restful sleep. It can also become a habit that you increase over time for the same effect. Sometimes you fall asleep immediately, but then you wake up a few hours later. Many people turn to alcohol to reduce stress; however, alcohol has similar taxing and addictive effects on the body like sugar. Alcohol acts like refined sugar in the body and has to be processed by the liver. See page 68, for more about the effects of sugar. If you drink alcohol, consider other soothing options to help you relax in the evenings.

* Change like the seasons. Different seasons pose various issues. I know it's tough to sleep when it's too hot or too cold. In the summer heat, it feels great to have a fan. That fan can turn stiff, hot, stale air into a comforting, cool breeze. In the winter and colder months, I love to place a hot water bottle on my belly. Not only does it keep me warm, it helps relax my muscles. I always sleep better with a hot water bottle on my belly.

* Alarms should be heard and not seen. Anxious glancing at the clock, followed by calculating and then ruminating about "when will I get to sleep" or "how many hours of sleep do I have left", are major causes of insomnia. If you have difficulty falling asleep, move your clock so you can hear the alarm but can't see the time.

* SHHHHH! There may be noises in your home that keep you from a deep sleep. It could be your partner's snoring or a roommate who stays up late watching TV. Consider earplugs, a white noise machine, or possibly sleeping in a different room.

* Sometimes you are just too tired and wired to read, write, or actually do anything but moan, groan and toss and turn at night. If you know sleep just isn't going to grace you at night, have a small, non-intrusive audio player that is stocked with encouraging audio books. If you are not going to sleep, then you may as well fill your mind with something positive. Plan ahead. You want soothing stories (NOT horror stories) to enter your subconscious at this precious time of night.

Write it Down to Figure it Out

Take just ONE day, and note all the ingredients you eat. This is best done on a day when you dine out or eat various packaged foods that you enjoy. See Food/Mood Journal in Blood-Sugarology on page 126.

Do this for just ONE day, and it will help you become aware of where you struggle with food and beverages.

I have said this over and over again throughout the book – remember you are NOT on a diet. It's time to investigate the ingredients and find healing Upgrades for foods that you love (possibly childhood or ancestral foods). Then learn how to create them in a way that will sustain your health and cravings.

Any sensitivity that you have to foods is a GOOD thing! WHY? Because it can wake you up to listen to the messages your body is trying to tell you. When you take medications for minor ailments, you mask the symptoms that work to give you a wake-up call. When you have a symptom, look for the root of the problem. **70% of your immune system is in your gut.** So when you have a gut ache, investigate why instead of masking it with an over-the-counter-medication. Instead, take natural steps such as drinking purified water, a stomach massage, digestive enzymes, or natural anti-inflammatories such as turmeric.

When you experience a symptom, get curious and investigate what causes your symptoms and begin to heal from the inside out. If the ailment is persistent, visit a holistic practitioner or herbalist to see if there are any natural remedies available. Over-the-counter medications have LOTS of side effects, even low suspecting antacids. Read the ingredients and side-effects.

You may be surprised to find things like sugar and artificial flavorings and colorings in chewable/drinkable items. Most of them have more side effects than benefits! Note: if you currently take prescription medication, please check with a medical practitioner before taking any natural supplements.

I worked with a client who had daily headaches so she did what most pharmacies or medical professionals tell you to do: take an over-the-counter pain reliever. Most of the pain relievers upset her stomach, and either made her constipated or have diarrhea. As we worked together, I encouraged her to keep a food and drink log for a few days. Looking at her food/mood journal, I immediately knew why she had headaches.

> #1 She was dehydrated (common source of headache).
> #2 She drank a lot of coffee (a stimulant that leads to dehydration).
> #3 She put artificial sweetener in her coffee (the biggest culprit).

Her overall food choices were decent so we focused on her drinks. I made some suggestions (see Beverage Upgrades in Chapter 6, page 142) for upgrading to an organic coffee and using organic green stevia powder with a little coconut sugar and coconut oil in it. I also suggested that she finish drinking her coffee before 11 am and increase her water intake and snacks in the afternoon. Within just one day of eliminating the artificial sweetener, her headache was significantly less.

The root of her headaches?
Artificial Sweeteners AND Dehydration

Within three days of drinking more water and having just one cup of organic coffee in the morning (ditching the artificial sweetener) **her headaches were gone!**

It's probable that if she never used the Food/Mood Journal that she would still have these 'mysterious' headaches. Writing down what you eat and drink can also help you get clear on where your ailments may stem from. Here are some baby steps to get you started with your ailment investigation.

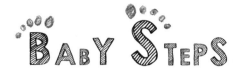

Jot down after lunch what you've eaten so far and what you crave:

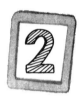

Write down what you eat/drink after each meal. Begin to notice and jot down how you feel. It can be as simple as: feel fine, feel bloated, feel tired, craving more, etc.

* **Dive into the Food/Mood Journal provided in Chapter 5 (page 126) and fill it out for just one week.**
* At the end of the week, see what you notice.
* What meals made you feel good and gave you energy?
* Which ones left you with undesirable symptoms?
* Are you drinking enough water?
* What are your sleep patterns?
* How are your bowel movements?

Stress Relief

"Nicole really gets the mindset of a life of food struggles, having gone through some herself. That really comes across, and you feel like you've got a partner in your journey that understands your thoughts and behaviors regarding food. I'm someone who doesn't like to be told what to do, so the traditional "you need to eat more vegetables and exercise" attitude turns me off. Nicole probes and challenges you to ask yourself questions and to figure out solutions that work for YOU, not others.

She also helped me to see that stress is a huge impact on our hormones and that stress isn't "big stuff" (death, loss of job, divorce, etc.) but rather an accumulation of small, daily stresses that aren't managed; and that we need to find ways to be aware in the moment instead of spinning off into stressful thinking. I also loved her idea of "Upgrades". It's not about stopping to eat chocolate (or whatever) cold turkey, it's about taking small steps to get to where you want to be. So instead of the candy bar you go for chocolate that is not processed, or dark chocolate. You get lots of information to help you understand what's going on with your hormones, but also practical steps to make changes that will have a positive, lasting impact in your life."
– Tina C, Virginia

Stress can create overwhelming feelings of anxiety, hopelessness, and sometimes depression. Often many people look for a quick fix such as numbing out on certain foods, alcohol, or drugs. Many turn to TV or entertainment as a companion and as a way to relax and tune-out. If this is true for you, begin to find ways that you can reduce stress in your life. Many people are often surprised that as they Upgrade their foods and release the Franken-ingredients their stress reduces as well. Find the baby steps that work for you and know that the more you Upgrade your food, the more you automatically Upgrade your life!

Become more focused, centered, and calmer by releasing stress.

Take a deep breath

Think about how you would be without your senses, especially your ability to breathe. My grandmother had emphysema. She struggled for every breath. It was exhausting being around her. But now when I remember to breathe, I breathe for her (as I used to pretend to do). If she got upset, I'd put my hand on her back (which she loved) and sat by her quietly. I'd say, "I'm going to breathe for you now." This made her chuckle, but it also helped her slow down and focus on her breathing for a few moments.

Breathing brings you into to the present moment and creates awareness with what's going on with your body. By taking slow deep breaths, this allows you to truly assess the situation and see the real picture.

Benefits: MORE oxygen to your brain allows you to move into problem-solving mode rather than swirling in the problem. By taking a deep breath, it can help lower your blood pressure and give you an overall feeling of calmness and relaxation.

"Breathing in, I calm my body. Breathing out, I smile.
Dwelling in the present moment, I know this is a wonderful moment."
– Thich Nhat Hahn, Being Peace

Meditation

You don't have to become a yogi or a monk to learn how to meditate or become mindful. A lot of research has gone into how meditation and mindfulness can bring you a sense of calm, clarity, and positive health benefits. Just five minutes a day of a meditative or mindful activity can help you reap these benefits. If you feel anxious or stressed, meditation/mindfulness alone can help you more than anything.

If you have never meditated before. Begin by sitting comfortably either on the floor of in a chair. Sit up tall and take a deep breath. Begin to notice your body and your surroundings. Then, close your eyes, breathe normally and begin to notice any sensation in your body. Stay here as long as it is comfortable and open your eyes when you are ready. Believe it or not, that was a meditation.

Moving Meditation

Meditation can help increase awareness of your cravings and food patterns. Meditation is that place where you feel connected. It is that space or mindset where you know you are not alone - either silently or loudly. I feel it every time I see the ocean, the forest, a beautiful landscape, or in the thick of a project. Where is your 'feel good place'?

Some people want to meditate but say "I can't sit still". There are many ways to meditate. For instance, Walking Meditation is where you walk very slowly, with intention and notice each movement in your body. For some their meditation is working on a project or "being in the zone". For some, it's being in nature, gazing up into the stars, or watching the clouds pass by. Some people find a natural meditative state while sitting in the park, looking at the ocean or watching the river flow. Meditation can be any activity or inactivity where you are aware of your surroundings, your breath, and have a sense of being present.

"The thing about meditation is: you become more and more you."
- David Lynch

What is YOUR moving meditation?

Stretch Breaks

- Take a short walk around the block.
- Turn on music and dance out your stress.
- Every 30 minutes, get up and take a one minute stretch break, and a few deep breaths.

With any of these stretches begin with doing one, check in with your body, and if the stretch feels good to you repeat each one 3-5 times. Until they feel comfortable, first go through these movements breathing naturally. When ready, inhale a deeper breath that connects with the movement.

Gentle Yoga - Standing Stretch

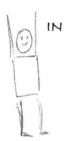 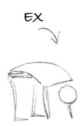

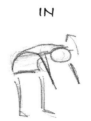 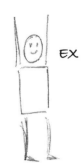

Stand up and reach your hands over your head and take a deep breath in.

On EXHALE, begin to reach down towards your toes.

Stay bent over for a few moments and continue to breathe easily.

When you are ready, slowly rise back up to standing on the INHALE.

Sitting Twist

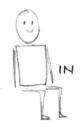 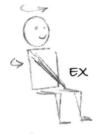 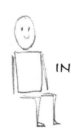 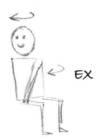 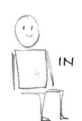

Sit up tall in your chair with both feet on the ground.

Look to your left Place right hand on left leg. Lengthen spine by sitting up tall and then twist to the left on EXHALE.

On INHALE, come back to center. Take a deep breath at center, sitting up tall.

Look to your right, place left hand on right leg. Lengthen spine by sitting up tall, then twist to the right on EXHALE.

On INHALE, come back to center.

Sitting Forward Fold

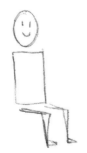 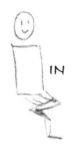 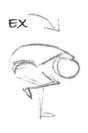 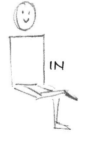 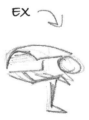 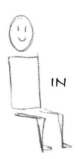

Sitting in your chair, sit up tall and take a deep breath.

Place your left ankle above your right knee.

Breathe in and sit up tall (this may be enough of a stretch if so, stay here and breathe).

Otherwise, exhale and gently begin to lean forward until you feel the stretch.

Breathe into it. INHALE as you come back to center.

Sitting tall, release left leg back to the floor. Take a centering breath here. **Repeat other side.**

* IN = INhale
* EX = EXhale

Sitting Lateral Stretch

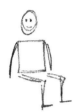 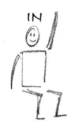 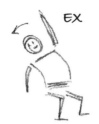 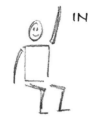 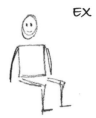

Sit up tall in your chair, both feet on the ground, and take a deep breath.

With your left hand, reach up towards your ear and above your head. Keep your back straight and long. INHALE here.

On EXHALE, begin to stretch laterally towards your RIGHT. Keep spine long so you don't slump into the stretch.

INHALE, come back to center.

EXHALE, bring left arm down.

Take a breath.

Repeat other side.

* IN = INhale
* EX = Exhale

Floor Stretches

Using a yoga mat or some kind of padding, move to the floor.
On the floor, come onto hands and knees.

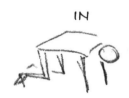 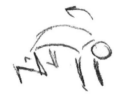 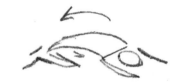

Place hands (elbows slightly bent) on the floor just under your shoulders.
Keep knees on the floor hips-width apart.
INHALE Table pose (hands and knees).

EXHALE and let your hips move back towards the floor/towards your hips.

Hands stay where they are.

Stretch arms stretch forward, hips towards the heels.
Repeat: INHALE Table pose (hands and knees).
EXHALE child's pose (hips to heels).
Repeat 5-6 times.

Gentle Twist

If you have any back issues, make sure you okay this movement with your doctor.
Lay on your back and take a deep breath in.

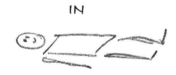 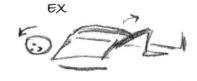

Bring your LEFT hand down and your RIGHT knee up until they meet.
With an EXHALE, place your left hand on your right knee and guide that right knee over to the left side of your body.

Look to your right.
Breathe into the twist.
Gently come out of the twist.
Take a breath at center.
Then twist and breathe in the other direction.

Back to Center - Knees To Chest

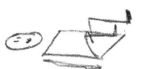
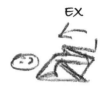
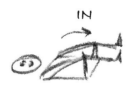

Bring your knees into your chest.

Place your hands on your knees (fingers towards your toes).

On the EXHALE, bring knees into your chest.

INHALE, let your knees fall out the length of your arms. Repeat a few times.

Legs Up The Wall

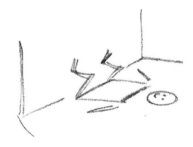
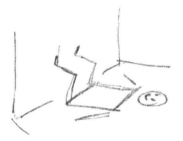
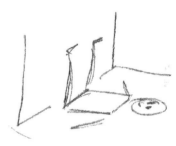
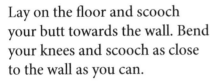

Lay on the floor and scooch your butt towards the wall. Bend your knees and scooch as close to the wall as you can.

Gently start to walk your legs up the wall until comfortable.

Lay here for a few minutes, and take a few deep breaths.

Benefits: Appropriate movement brings about the feel-good chemicals in your body. Movement increases oxygen flow which reduces stress. Exercise helps elevate your mood, increases sleep and create MORE energy. You gotta spend to receive.

Passion

What's your passion? Are you doing something every day that feeds your passions? What is that ONE positive thing in your life -something creative that puts you in 'the zone'? You know that place where you are engulfed in your project and hours and hours go by and you are just in your bliss? What is that place? I know you think you are too busy and don't have time for your passion, but the reason is you don't MAKE time for it. If you engage in mindless activities (surfing the internet, watching TV, etc.), you waste precious time that could be spent on your passion. And the less time you spend on what you are passionate about, the more time you may tend to spend on mindless activities.

Helpful tip:

* Dedicate just 10 minutes every day in the morning towards something you love.
* I've suggested this to various clients throughout the years and it has made an impressionable difference in their lives when they take this 10 minute morning ritual to heart.

A friend of mine woke at 5 am so that he had time to write every morning before going to work. With this ritual, he found he was able to complete his book of short stories within three months. He commented on how it made his entire day better by getting up first thing to write his book before heading out to his job. He said that not only was his day better, but he found that he had ideas during the day that he would jot down. He also became so inspired that sometimes he would come home at night after work and write (he rarely had the energy for this before starting his morning ritual). Before taking on this ritual, he was convinced he'd never finish his book. With this morning ritual, he DID finish his book!

I resisted this for some time as well. Once I began to put my passions first in the morning, it set the tone of my day. On mornings where I first checked e-mail, it seemed to take me hours to get into the groove. On mornings where writing (or art) is the first thing I do, my entire day has a more productive flow.

Give it a try for one week and see what works for you. Begin with just 5 minutes dedicated towards something you know will improve your day. It can be a walk, a few stretches, engaging in a favorite sport or activity. Take a few minutes to write, paint, draw, craft, etc.

Shake Shake Shake

Animals know how to release themselves of stress and trauma by shaking. When an animal encounters a stressful or life-threatening event, they begin to shake or they will freeze and then shake once danger has passed. They do this naturally. Once their episode of shaking stops, they are usually relieved of the stress or trauma. We humans can learn a lot by observing animals.

Over the years, I've adopted this practice of shaking. If any kind of stressful or traumatic event happens, I will go where I feel safe and/or alone and begin to shake with my entire body. I'll let sounds come out and do anything from tremble to full out shaking. Sometimes that's not enough and I need to add in auditory sounds and purposely push out as much air as possible, which forces me to take in deeper breaths. I always feel better after shaking.

Give shaking a try the next time something triggers you, stresses you, or even small traumas such as being cut off while driving. In ANY close call while driving, I'll find the safest way to pull over as soon as I can. If it's on the freeway I'll wait until I can get off the freeway. Then I'll sit in the car, shake, tremble, and sometimes talk or yell out my fears. When I feel complete, I'll then continue with my travels. This above all else has helped me manage stress and trauma.

Scream and Shout About It!

Find a safe place, grab a pillow and scream into it! My favorite place is in the car and I just let it out. Sometimes crying comes after I scream and that's okay. Once I begin to feel frustration, I do my best to be alone and release that primal scream. Notice children and their tantrums… if they are allowed to scream it out, they will eventually calm down and then move onto the next thing. If only you, as an adult, could just lie down in the grocery store and have a fit without the psych ward being called. We all need to let it out sometimes, but just don't let it out on other people. When you build up tension, anger and stress inside (without releasing it in healthy ways), you may start to take it out on other people. If you allow yourself to have 'secret' tantrums, you will able to move on, and let it go.

Your furry friends

Animals are simple creatures and a fine example of how to enjoy life. I know there are some neurotic animal breeds out there, but find an animal that doesn't feel threatened. Just hang out with them and observe them. How do they breathe? Notice how even in a calm state most animals breathe deeply. Animals want food, love, exercise, and rest. If you need to get out and walk more, dogs are amazing companions. If you don't have time to take care of an animal or are out and about most of the day, most cats are pretty self-reliant. Even something like having fish can enhance your life. Having something to take care of such as a pet or even a plant can bring more fulfillment and meaning into your life.

Laugh

Don't be afraid to laugh at yourself. Find something funny – it can be a memory, a cartoon, or anything that makes you smile. I have a Persian cat and she is hilarious to me. I don't need to go very far to add humor to my life on a daily basis. So what works for you? If you love to watch shows, pick a show that's sweet and funny and makes you feel good.

Sing your favorite song

Singing lifts depression and raises your spirits. Turn on positive music that you love and play that stuff loud and proud! Take singing and dancing breaks throughout your day. Find someplace to be alone (if you don't want others to hear), and then sing and act out the song. Don't worry about what others think. Imagine you are a performer and you have to practice every day! This helps prepare you for your daily performance of showing up as your best (and not your most stressed).

It's all about the...

This book is about food yet it's not ALL about food. It's all connected. Sugars and processed foods drain your energy and increase stress. Keep snacks with you and set alarms to remind you to eat them. When your blood sugar drops too low from not having enough fuel, this creates stress. Many people make their biggest mistakes (and have the most far out arguments) when their blood sugar drops too low. Don't get caught with low blood sugar – REMEMBER to always have snacks on hand. See Snacks in Chapter 5 (page 114) and Healing Foods in Chapter 7 (page 161).

Talk to someone positive

Find a confidante/friend or family member who inspires you. If you don't have this person in your life, print out a picture of your idol and have an 'out loud' conversation with them. Ask out loud: What would Oprah (insert favorite inspirational person) do? Then listen for your answer or just keep talking until you feel resolved!

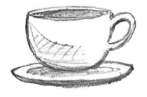

Unplug and get connected with nature and real people

Turn off the gadgets, explore nature, and find ways to feel connected. Talk to a friend or loved one that inspires you, or sit with a dog, cat, or baby. Look at the wonderment of the world with new, fresh child-like eyes. Social media can be a false sense of connection if you don't have nature and real time with people. If your entire network is via the computer or phone, then this may be the very reason you feel lonely and dis-connected. It's tempting and so easy to be alone with gadgets these days. A true sense of feeling good is when we are in nature and/or around people and community that inspire you and help you see the best in yourself and others.

Finance$

This is a major stressor for most people! Car and financial troubles get me fired up every time, so I really have to work on this. Spend some time figuring out your personal budget. A monthly plan is the best way to prepare and keep track of your finances, instead of letting them surprise you each time you get a bill or have a new expense. There are lots of free resources online for financial assistance and suggestions on how to keep a budget.

Here are some ways to help keep your finances on track:

*   Create a budget and stick to it.

*   If more money goes out than comes in, see where you can trim in order to stay within budget.

*   If you need to earn money, think of fun, interesting ways to make extra income. Take the passions that you have and turn them into a money-making opportunity. Do you love art? Maybe you could work at a local art gallery or art store. Do you love books? Look for a part time-job at a book store or library. Do you love cars? Check out part-time jobs at a mechanics/car shop. Do you love TV? Find a part- time job at an electronics store. Turn your hobbies into part-time jobs.

*   Bring in more of the things that you love to do with your life, and there will be more of your life that you will love and enjoy.

Delegate Your Issues

Have more money than time and feeling stressed? Then delegate the things you need to do. For example, pay to have your house cleaned or your laundry done. If you have more time than money, don't waste your time in front of the TV. Find a part-time job that you love (and feeds your passions) and go from there. Even if you are paid minimum wage, see it as a volunteer opportunity and a gift. It's a good opportunity to get paid to learn or be around what you love to do.

*"It's none of my business what people say of me and think of me.
I am what I am and I do what I do. I expect nothing and accept everything.
And it makes life so much easier" – Anthony Hopkins*

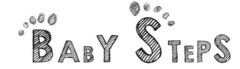

BABY STEPS

Write down 3 things from Wellnessology that are interested in doing daily.

1.

2.

3.

Start with #1 for 5 minutes today.
If you feel like it or have the time, incorporate 5 minutes of #2 and/or #3

After you try out 1-3 of your top three, pick just ONE to do consistently for one week. Write it down on your calendar that you will do this activity for just 5 minutes. Write down the time you will do this. Keep in mind that it's just 5 minutes. This way it does not feel overwhelming, but if you decide to go longer that's great. If you stick with 5 minutes, you will be successful.

After giving your best to one of the above for 5 minutes every day, see if there is another activity you can incorporate for just 5 minutes per day. Again, only commit to 5 minutes (if you go longer, great). Leave it open-ended so that you feel inspired by the 5 minutes. 30 minutes can easily get pushed off but 5 minutes is very do-able.

Gratitude

Write down three things you are grateful for when you start to feel stressed or anxious. Look at your problems with perspective. Know that there is ALWAYS a solution. Keep a gratitude journal with you. It can be a small pad of paper that you write on when things seem bleak, or jot down your thoughts when you feel really amazing. Write down ALL of your successes. Then go through each one and allow yourself to really experience what's going well for you. Practice focusing on what's going well and you will find that more things go well for you.

"There is always something to be grateful for."
– Mother Teresa

Movement & Exercise

Making time for movement in your life gives you more energy and MORE time! You will sleep better and experience LESS fatigue. After a while, my clients start to realize that movement IS their magic pill. Exercise may just be the closest thing to that magic pill that we all want.

Here's your Magic Movement Pill = **Movement that works WITH YOUR body!** Stop comparing yourself with others when it comes to exercise. You are awesomely YOU! You are the only YOU, so be YOU! Just the word "exercise" can deter you from being physically active. Do you picture a sweaty gym, feeling uncomfortable, or aches and pain resulting from exercise? But what if your exercise was fun? Something that you DO enjoy? Something that feels easy? Something that you are willing to do in SMALL amounts every day?

For the longest time, I rebelled against movement as I grew up in a very sports-related and movement-intense family. I was also clumsy and injured myself with some of the simplest things. I broke my ankle falling off a bike. Heck, I even broke that same ankle again getting up from a lawn chair, while all the other kids ran around playing. My parents didn't believe me that day at the pool. It wasn't until my ankle was double the size and purple the next morning that they took me to the ER. I fell down a lot. I hated the smell of the gym and I quit karate after breaking my wrist (not in karate practice, but from falling off a desk in school). When I found a gentle form of yoga and dance, it felt like coming home. Yoga and dance moved my body in simple, easy ways full of awareness and pleasure. I had to find the right movement for me! I also love Qigong and Tai Chi.

My morning routine is now a non-negotiable for me. It gets done every morning, BEFORE checking any e-mail or internet or electronic anything! I created a checklist/calendar for myself. It has been amazing to see how I struggled to get through day one and day two to making it through weeks and months. Where does the time go? It goes fast whether you exercise or not, and it feels great to look back at all my check marks and hearts on the calendar representing the days I've exercised. There are some amazing tools you can re-adopt from your kindergarten years. We all love to see ourselves progress so let's bring back the star charts!

Benefits of Movement

* Increases your ability to release weight
* Reduces depression and anxiety, even better than anti-depressants!
* Helps with blood sugar regulation - important for any blood sugar issues such as: pre-diabetes, hypoglycemia, Type II diabetes, etc.
* Natural pick-me up. When you feel tired, a walk can help you more than a cup of coffee!
* Relieves pain - when doing appropriate movement and stretches
* Improves brain function and memory
* Enhances the immune system

Movement Options

* Walking (or walk around during TV commercials)
* Bicycling
* Gardening
* Stretching
* Swimming
* Exercising at a gym
* Gentle movement classes (i.e. Yoga, Dance, Nia, Tai Chi, Qigong, etc.)
* Exercise video games & online videos
* Roll around on the floor & just have fun!

Join a walking group or a gentle movement class…the hardest part is getting there! When you start exercising with a friend or a group, it's always easier. Every walk I take with someone usually lasts longer than walking by myself! Have a walk-n'-talk or take a walk or stretch meeting with co-workers. The next time you want to sit and chat with someone, take that chat from the table to the sidewalk!

Another great way to add movement to your day is to join a partner or group dance class. Not only will it get you moving, but it helps you meet other supportive people too! For all of you busy moms, try this new routine with your family. When you wake up in the morning, have everyone stretch or exercise WITH you. Not only will it benefit YOU, it benefits the entire family!

Add MORE movement to your day!

* Park just one parking space further than you normally would.
* Walk one more block to the bus stop or all the way to your destination.
* Get up from your desk every 30 minutes and walk to the door, hallway, or outside. This actually makes you more productive!
* Take a walk around the block.
* Take one more stroll around the fruits and veggies aisle when shopping.
* Find creative, fun, and feel-good chair, couch, or bed stretches that you enjoy.
* Do a mini-dance while waiting in line.
* Pace while you talk on the phone.

Simple, no-equipment exercises for your home and office:

* Use the furthest bathroom possible. Upstairs? Great! Take the stairs.
* Choose the stairs over the elevator.
* Eat lunch away from your desk and leave time for a 5-10 minute walk.
* Move your trashcan/printer/file cabinet further away from your desk to add more steps to your day.
* Step outside! Enjoy nature, breathe in some fresh air, and then return to work.
* Stand while you wait for the bus or train.
* Stand at the back of the room during a meeting to "stretch out".
* Offer to go to co-workers' offices for meetings.
* Walk to your co-worker's office instead of e-mailing them.
* Walking or fostering a dog is an excellent way to ensure walks.

The above accumulated movements can be more beneficial than going to the gym once a week!

Find what works for you and DO it - make it a non-negotiable!

What word works for you instead of exercise?
i.e. movement, motion, easy, etc. (make up one that suits you)

Words I like that encourage me to move my body _____

Songs that inspire me to move _____

Movement Worries

Movement can bring up many different emotions. Many people, like myself, have rebelled against exercise due to the stigmas associated with it so let's take a looksee at some of this hogwash that we tell ourselves!

1. "No Pain, No Gain"

Yeah - this one is a doozy! It works for a certain kind of athletic personality, but for those of us who avoid movement that causes pain, this just keeps us from exercising. "No pain, no gain" again taps into that perfectionism. What if we change it to: do it YOUR way to a no-pain movement routine with all the gain! OR Yes Gain, No Pain or appropriate movement for me looks easy and fun.

My new motto of feeling positive towards my body's appropriate movement is_____

2. But you have to be thin to exercise!

This was a strong belief of mine for a long time. I thought that once I lose the weight then I'll be more inspired to exercise. The problem is that the two go hand-in-hand. Eating real foods with real nutrients, along with an easy movement plan, creates a synergy that helps us reach our body positive goals.

The perfect movement for my body right now is _____

I'm not a fan of the gym. I don't like all of the hassle, the blaring TV's or the smell of it. The gym is not the only place to move! If you don't like going to a gym, there are many options available to you (see Movement Options on page 217). Every time you move that's a good thing. Find movement that YOU enjoy and do it just a little bit every day.

Movement I enjoy is _____

3. But I'll get hurt!

Another thing about exercise that many people don't talk about is the potential for injury. For someone like me who had many injuries as a young person, it makes double sense that I would be very cautious of exercise. So if you have some fears about exercise and injury, then it's time to shift your thoughts about exercising. Think of exercise/movement as healing instead of potentially harmful. Running may not be an appropriate form of exercise for someone who's overweight, or with any knee, back, ankle or foot issues. Why? Because it could create more injury, and injury creates more fear of movement. Fear of movement creates more sedentary days… and that creates more illness, aches, and pains in our bodies. Do any movement that YOU enjoy!

Appropriate movement that's a good fit for you can actually eliminate pain. If you experience lower body pain then work with your upper body. Swimming in a pool (hydrotherapy) is also helpful for severe pain. If you don't want to participate in intense exercise, try gentle stretches in the bed, bath or shower (this might be a better alternative for your body).

Movement that is safe for me today is _____

4. I don't have the energy/ I'm too tired

Start slowly. Try movement that feels good to you, and something that is fun. Put on music that moves you to dance or walk around a beautiful place and it won't feel like exercise.

Movement that is ease for me today is _____

5. I don't have the time

This comes from some of the above issues. You DO have 5 minutes each and every day to move your body in some way. You DO!

Look at your day and think about when you can carve out 5 minutes each day for movement that's enjoyable and is good for your body right now_____

Weight release

Do you have excess weight you'd like to release? The main focus here is on health and nourishment instead of restrictions, diets, guilt and deprivation. As you may have experienced in the past with diets, they only last so long before things like deprivation, temptation, stress, trauma, holidays, special events, etc. happen.

Natural weight release happens when certain things are aligned:
* Nourishing foods are eaten
* Stress is low
* Digestion is working
* Getting enough quality sleep
* Engaged in activities you are passionate about
* A sense of belonging or community
* Feeling in alignment with how you live your life

At first, this may seem like a tall order. The suggestions you find within Upgradeology all point in the direction of these alignments. Notice that the bulk of this book is about nourishing sources of food.

❋ Without healing and nourishing foods, it's nearly impossible to relieve your body of stress and have adequate digestive health.

❋ With high stress and poor digestion, it's difficult to get quality sleep or engage fully in the activities that you are passionate about.

❋ Without fully engaging in the things you love, it's difficult to feel that you are in alignment with the life you want to lead.

This brings us back to the food. I believe that **by Upgrading your food, you will be able to revive your health, increase digestion, release unnecessary stresses and as a result, begin to release excess weight... slowly.** Releasing weight slowly is more effective. Why? Because if you eat foods you enjoy and slowly release the weight at the same time, you are **more** likely to keep it off. Upgrading your food and **enjoying** your Upgrades can change your entire life for the positive.

Some things to keep in mind about Weight Release:

Do you let your scale determine how you feel about yourself? Geene Roth said it best: *"Scales are for fish."* I know the scale is tempting, but if the scale tips a high number - do you feel bad about yourself? I don't own a scale, because I don't want to let it determine if I feel good or bad about myself that day. If you can't resist the scale, then I'd recommend donating it. Get that scale out of your house so that it won't tempt you. **Focus on how you FEEL, not some fakakta** (useless/crappy) **number on the Scale!**

Self-Talk or Self-Sabotage?

Most affirmations just don't cut it. **If you don't believe the affirmation, then your mind says "LIAR!"** It can *seem* like the best affirmation in the world, but if you don't truly believe it, then your mind only knows that you are lying to it. **Let your self-talk be true!** Let your self-talk be supportive, NOT abusive. Abusive self-talk will lead you right back into the unhealthy habits. **Supportive self-talk will guide you to understand your patterns and ultimately lead you to healing and nourishing inclinations.**

Instead of: *I am the perfect weight*, OR *I am naturally thin*, OR *I lose weight easily and effortlessly...*

Let it be: **I DESIRE to be healthy**
or **I DESIRE to accept myself and my weight as it is today**
or **I WANT to create nourishing habits that heal my body, mind and spirit**, etc...

This is language that your mind can say **"Ah yes... she is telling me the truth, this IS what I desire."** Give it a try!

Old fakakta (useless/crappy) **Affirmation:**

New Truthful, Kind & Believable Affirmation:

If you have a substantial amount of weight to release, set your focus towards nourishing habits. **Set your intention to release the number and embody your wellbeing. Why?** As you well know with diets, **if weight comes off quickly then you usually gain it back even quicker.** It's also proven that the slower you release the weight and adopt nurturing habits, **the easier it will be to maintain that weight release.** Do what you can to release that expectation of dropping 10 pounds in 20 days to fit into that party dress! Begin to accept that this is a **new** and **nourishing** way to approach your health. This helps you to create a future filled with healing instead of the unhealthy, continual yo-yo dieting and negative self-judgment.

> **Self-Acceptance and Self-Kindness will give you MORE happiness than you ever imagined possible. Self-Kindness is MORE beautiful and MORE fulfilling than that 'ideal' body could ever be.**

Keep it Simple!

* Instead of beating yourself up, begin to incorporate self-acceptance and self-kindness. Allow yourself to move into what you **CAN** do today! Begin **one little healing routine** that will start or continue your journey.

* **Start SMALL! Do ONE thing**: For example: *Today I will drink 64 ounces of purified water.* Once you've got that down, THEN add in something else.

* **What is your One SMALL Thing?** Write it here:

Blood Sugar Stabilization

Start with breakfast (See Breakfast section on page 158). If you skip breakfast and are hungry all day, then at night there will be no stopping you because you've gone over the tipping point. Even if you don't feel hungry at breakfast, get into the habit of eating nourishing food in the morning.

If you tend to eat a lot of food at night, try this for a week: Eat an Upgraded breakfast at least 1 hour upon rising. Eat every 2 – 3 hours. See what this does for your evening munchies.

Sample Schedule
*   7:00 am – Breakfast
*   12:30 pm – Lunch
*   7:00 pm – Dinner
*   10:00 am – Snack
*   3:30 pm – Snack
*   9:00 pm - Snack

Eat your dinner at least three hours before going to bed. Going to sleep on a full stomach makes your body work overtime at night. If you have difficulty with curbing the evening munchies check in to make sure you are eating enough food during the day. A light snack before bed such as a handful of almonds, nuts or seeds can sometimes assist with being able to get to sleep. Foods that are high in magnesium will have this effect.

Drink warm comforting fluids like Chamomile Tea or Golden Milk in the evening.

Move first thing in the morning. Refer to Movement Options.

Keep food ingredients clean, eat nourishing quality fats, and snacks (see Snacks page 114 & Gotta Go Bag page 118). The more consistent your blood sugar is throughout the day, the better you will feel during the evening. Nourishing fats can help assist mind clarity and weight release. Fat-free/non-fat foods are mostly toxic and lead to cravings for MORE foods.

Upgrade from diet and processed foods! These frankenfoods just confuse your body's metabolism and have been PROVEN to cause weight gain. It's sad but true.

All calories are NOT the same. The calories in a diet frozen entrée are not the same as calories from a freshly prepared Upgraded meal. 100 calories of toxic diet pudding is NOT the same as 100 calories from a nourishing avocado. So many diets are calorie focused, and that's why there are so many 'diet foods' on the market. Choose Upgraded foods and see the difference yourself. You will notice more satisfaction, less cravings, and an easier way to release the weight and keep it off.

Note: Fasting and detox cleanses send the body into starvation mode. A few years ago, I did over 7 fasts within an 18 month period. I lost 10-20 lbs in a short amount of time and then gained it back almost immediately. This really took a toll on my body and self-esteem. With each fast, the weight came back quicker and quicker. No matter how I planned, measured out my food, slowly came off the fast, it didn't matter. The moment I started eating again, the cravings and binge eating seemed never ending. Someone like me with a history of eating disorders is a terrible candidate for fasting and detoxes, because fasting only triggers the eating disorder and deprivation. I'd go from the anorexic mentality of wanting to fast forever to the inability to stop eating once I started.

Release the pressure of Diets, Harsh Detoxes and Fasting! They all lead to deprivation and create cravings! Eating Upgraded foods is a simple, kind and nourishing detox for your body. JUST getting away from toxic foods is a natural and effective detox if your current food plan includes frankenfoods.

If diets and fasts have not worked for you in the past, why do we keep thinking that the next one will be the solution? Stress = increases cortisol production = taxes your body and prompts your body to hold onto weight.

Diets, fasts, and extreme detox protocols create stress on the body. As a result, the amount of cortisol in our body increases. This is the reason we gain weight so quickly after coming off a diet, fast or detox. We have snapped the rubber band from restriction to overdoing it. I have struggled with weight for as long as I can remember. I've learned that what works for me is to eat nourishing, clean food, start with breakfast, have nourishing snacks, and make sure I eat a good dinner so that I don't feel hungry at night. Many of my clients find that their cravings begin to lessen when following these simple ideas. Upgrade, make sure your food tastes good, and don't go more than 3 hours during the day without eating. See more about snacks and blood sugar stabilization on page 114.

"I find that when we really love and accept and approve of ourselves exactly as we are, then everything in life works."
- Louise L. Hay

How to Eat: Chewing & Digestion

Do you eat slowly or fast? Do you focus on your food while eating or are you multi-tasking? Eating food too quickly, without chewing, leads to increased stress, compromised digestion, and increased cravings. The less you pay attention to your food, the more food you are bound to eat.

Ever notice how a lot of snack food disappears when you watch a movie or TV? Did you eat meals while working, watching TV, driving or engaged in other activities? After that meal or snack, do you feel full but still want more food? Are you aware that you eat MORE when you don't pay attention to the food you are eating? The more you pay attention to your food, the more satisfying it becomes. The more we multi-task while eating (I still eat and work more than I'd like to admit) the less satisfying our meal becomes and we can often find ourselves wanting more food.

The MORE you pay attention while eating and chew your food, the more you break down the food, and it becomes easier to digest. The MORE you chew your food, the more saliva is produced. Saliva contains enzymes that help you digest your food. Therefore, the MORE you chew your food, more saliva is produced, which creates a smoother and more complete digestion of the food you are eating.

At your next meal or snack, begin to notice how you eat. Do you sit at a park bench, enjoy the scenery, chew your food slowly, and enjoy every bite? Are you aware of ALL the tastes and textures in your food?

A client was a binge eater so I suggested that **the next time she went for her 'binge' foods to slow down, and allow herself to enjoy each and every bite.** I explained that either way she is going to eat it, right? She agreed and decided to test this out.

223

If you hate on yourself while eating your food, and gobble it down without chewing, it won't digest well. HOWEVER, if you chew it and enjoy every single bite, even if the ingredients are toxic for you, the whole situation is LESS toxic IF there is a good amount of digestion involved. If you are going to eat it, then you may as well enjoy it and be able to assimilate it as best you can!

At first, my client thought it was an absurd exercise. However, when she slowed down to eat her 'binge' food she found it didn't even taste that good. The same thing happens with 'healthy' food. If someone feels angry and eats a carrot (or any other nutritious food), then the food will not assimilate as well compared to eating it and chewing it completely when feeling calm.

Prepare for Eating

Try out some of these ideas to increase chewing, digestibility, and the pleasure of your food.

* Turn off all distractions for at least one meal or snack per day.
* Find a quiet, relaxing place to eat (i.e. at the table, park, or a soothing environment).
* Play soft, calming music, light a candle, or just listen to the sounds in nature.
* Think about where your food came from and give thanks and/or say a prayer.

Stay Present
* Pay attention to the food you eat.
* Eat one bite at a time.
* Place your food or eating utensil on the plate in between bites.
* Very important: stay present in the moment and eat with intention.

At the End of the Meal
* Be grateful for the food you just ate.
* Take some quiet time to relax. This gives your body and mind the time to digest the meal.
* Go for a walk outside.

Write down what stuck out for you:

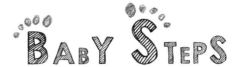

 Begin to notice when and where you eat. Do you eat in front of the TV, at work, in the car, on the go? Track in your Food/Mood Journal, page 126.

 Make a conscious effort to eat just one snack, or a portion of one meal without distractions.

Example: I had a client who always watched TV while eating dinner. The compromise was that he would sit at the table, take three bites of his dinner, chew it slowly, and then returned to watching TV. EVERY little step is a step towards awareness; therefore, you create SUCCESS! Don't knock it! Those three bites were probably the most nourishing part of his meal!

 **Make a ritual with just one meal or snack and eat it with mindful awareness.** Make it work for you (i.e. sit at your kitchen table, in the park, in the yard, etc.)

Take some time to reflect on your whole body wellness. Pick and choose the baby steps that work for you. Be gentle with yourself and at the same time push yourself to incorporate the passions that make you feel supported and happy. Involving yourself in more of the things that make you feel good, will inspire you to cultivate more of the things that truly support you.

Becoming more aware of the things that are going well in your life.

Incorporating gratitude for what is, and becoming clear on what you DO want will help propel you towards happiness. You'll reach far more success with the Upgrade Process if you slowly take baby steps that nourish your WHOLE self – physically, emotionally and spiritually.

Sugar & Food Addiction

More and more information and studies are coming out to prove that sugar is an addictive substance. As I mentioned in Chapter 4, it's as addictive as drugs and alcohol for certain people. Not everyone has addictive tendencies, but many people struggle with food addictions and eating disorders every day. Food, unlike drugs and alcohol, is essential for life. I absolutely identify as a food and sugar addict. With this knowledge I have sought out how to eat without being triggered by the foods I'm eating. I personally have to completely stay away from refined sugar, processed and artificial foods.

To recap what I discussed in Chapter 4, it takes about 2 weeks to get sugar out of our system. Just as it takes time for a drug addict or alcoholic to detox. I bring this up because it just might be the key factor for you as well. Do you struggle with not being able to stop eating a particular food once you have it or constantly battle with cravings? It could be that something in your food is triggering this response.

In the Sweetology section (pages 83-85), I list numerous sweeteners that are natural and delicious. Some people do very well on these Upgraded Sweeteners, but for others it may still trigger their sugar and food addictions tendencies. If you find that you are triggered by these Upgraded Sweeteners (i.e. increases cravings, you can't stop eating or thinking about the item, leads you back into the frankenfoods, etc.) then you may want to experiment with using natural fruits, sweet vegetables and/or organic stevia as your primary source of sweetness. The Upgraded Sweeteners listed are 100% MORE natural and healthier than ANY of the refined and artificial sugars. It's important to experiment with these Upgraded Sweeteners if you tend to crave and give into sugary foods. Why? Because if you 'fall off the wagon' and have an Upgraded alternative then you are not harming your body as much as you would by going back to refined, artificial sweeteners. It's a fine line when cravings and addictions are involved.

Many people might look at my food plan and ask "What kind of diet are you on"? To the world of 'normal eaters', I have a very restrictive food plan. Don't think that I'm not often tempted by what I no longer eat. However, I know that these foods will make me feel worse, never better. With a lot of work and trial and error over the years, it's just crystal clear to me what I do and do not eat. If I were to think of my food plan as a diet, I would fall off the wagon, again, and again, and again. However, when I think of my food plan as a way of life, as a way to keep me healthy and energized, it works and I'm satisfied by it!

When I take the foods that nourish me and get VERY CREATIVE with them, then I don't feel deprived. This is the essence of this book: **take the foods you know are nourishing for you and make them delicious and satisfying.** Without this key factor, it's a diet, and as we are all fully aware, a diet is only temporary. What I seek for you, my clients and myself is long term healing and the ability to be released from the addictive hold that sugar, gluten, refined, and processed frankenfoods hold over us. The problem isn't willpower, I KNOW the problem is in the toxic ingredients. I believe that the solution is in nourishing ingredients.

It is my hope that this book brings you awareness that there is a long-term solution to food-related inflammation, excess weight, diseases, and addictions. **That solution is to know your ingredients, and to know yourself well enough to choose what works and what doesn't work for you.** This takes time, patience, and the willingness to experiment. Within these pages are many tools you can use and alter to your specific needs. **Become clear on the ingredients that serve you well and the creativity to make them nourishing and satisfying to you.**

In Chapter 9 we discussed:
* The importance of restful sleep
* How journaling can assist you with your goals
* The importance of baby steps
* Stress Relief
* Meditation
* Moving Meditation
* Simple Stretches
* Shaking out trauma and fear
* Scream and shout about it, don't hold it in - the controlled tantrums!
* Furry Friends
* How Laughing, singing and dancing will lift your spirits
* Knowing that it's not about the food, but it's not - not about the food either.
* Positive influences in your life
* The importance of unplugging the gadgets and plugging into nature
* Budgets, organization and delegation
* The abundance of gratitude
* Body positive and weight release
* Chewing and Digestion
* Sugar and Food Addiction

The final chapter is a quick reference and detailed summary of Upgradeology. This is a great resource to glance at once a week to see which baby steps you can re-commit to and move towards.

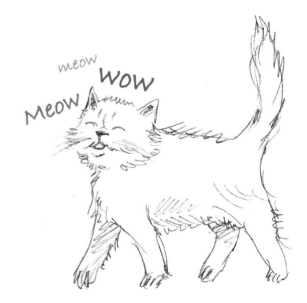

9.5 Summary
Baby Steps

Summary of Baby Steps
These will guide and help you throughout the Upgrade process

Get curious and take baby steps towards your health goals.
* Know that willpower is not something you are deficient in, it may be that you are deficient in the nutrients which won't allow you to stay away from the foods that may be harming you.
* Get curious! Learn what is in your food and what is truly causing your symptoms.
* Cultivate being grateful, the more you are grateful for, the more there is to BE grateful for.
* Write out the things you want and begin to take small action steps towards them.
* Think more about how to solve the problem, rather than begin stuck in the problem.

Honor your cravings, listen to them, investigate them and they will guide you to understanding their root messages.
* Notice our culture's obsession with instant gratification, and how much advertising goes into getting you addicted to refined and processed foods.
* Get curious about all of the medications and 'instant gratification' products on the market. What exactly does that next diet or diet pill promise you?
* Understand, within yourself, when you are hungry and when you eat due to stress or emotion, or if you are triggered by certain ingredients.

Drink Purified Water
* Look out for signs of dehydration and make drinking purified water a priority.

Become a Committed Label Reader
* Read EVERY label, every INGREDIENT and begin to understand what is in your food.
* Know the different names of sugar and become a food investigator/Ingredientologist.
* Don't let that unwanted sugar sneak in with a name you don't understand.

Upgrade from Artificial Sweeteners/Flavors/Colors and Chemicals
* All Artificial food-like products are Toxic! Some more than others.
* The Franken-ingredients INCREASE your appetite and create more and more cravings.
* Artificial sweeteners disturb your metabolism, can increase fat storage, and create dis-ease in your system.

Eat Naturally Sweet and Nurturing Foods
* Add in: Organic Fresh Sweet Vegetables & Fruits.
* Upgrade to: Organic hormone & antibiotic-free, pasture raised (not factory farmed) Proteins.
* Upgrade: White/Refined/Processed 'Fast Carbs' with Organic Whole Grains and Legumes known as 'Slow Carbs' or 'Complex Carbohydrates'.
* Find Upgraded alternatives for the refined and processed foods you love and crave.

UPGRADE

*   If you go 'Cold Turkey' from sugar, gluten, artificial and processed foods, this can lead to feelings of confusion and cravings. Transition to the Upgraded options first, so that your body and mind don't go into diet-mode.
*   Know what foods you crave and then find the cleanest Upgrade you can. If you desire something sweet, first try Upgraded Sweeteners, fruit or a sweet vegetable, and go from there.
*   Example: If you love chocolate, find an Upgraded chocolate or see Recipes Section.
*   Example: If you love crackers, find a gluten-free, artificial, and sugar-free cracker alternative or refer to Upgrades Chart. Get creative and make your own.
*   More and more people are becoming aware of the importance of clean and nourishing ingredients - therefore if you shop at a health food store you will continue to see products with cleaner and Upgraded ingredients. This is a win-win!

Appropriate Movement

*   Find out what's appropriate for your body type and activity level.
*   Create a movement routine that you LOVE and is enjoyable to YOU!
*   If you don't currently have a movement habit, begin with a 5 minute daily walk or stretching routine.

Restore with Adequate and Restful Sleep

*   If possible - get to sleep by 10 pm optimal (natural circadian rhythm).
*   Between 10 pm and Midnight is the most optimal, restorative sleeping time.
*   Get restful sleep naturally, using only natural herbs like Chamomile, Magnesium or Melatonin.

Reduce Stress

*   Find the best natural stress reducer for yourself .
*   Walking, Yoga, Meditation, Tai Chi, Dancing, Singing, Talking with an Inspirational Friend, Support.
*   Organize your time and learn to say NO to the things you don't want to do!

PASSION - Engage in something you love!

*   Make time DAILY for activities you are passionate about.
*   Make sure to do something you love, that is relaxing and fulfilling, every day.
*   If you enjoy crafts, but don't feel you have any time, give yourself 10 minutes every day to enjoy this activity. It's most beneficial if you can do it first thing in the morning.
*   As the day goes by, you may find more and more excuses as to why you don't have the time for the things that matter most to you.

Support and Help!

*   Do you think you can do this alone?
*   How many restrictive diets and torturing regimens have you attempted?
*   How many cookie-cutter diets have you tried that haven't worked?
*   Connect with me about how to create a bio-individual plan that works for you! www.Upgradeology.com or www.NicoleWhiteWellness.com

Recipes

Almond Biscotti 262
Almond Milk 234
Amaranth Veggie Patties 241
Apple Butter 248
Apple Cider Vinegar Tonic 31
Avocado & Kale Salad 255
Avocado Lemon Dill Dressing 253
Avocado Mushroom Sauce 252
Baby Food 261
Banana "Ice Cream" 259
Basic Vegetable Broth 240
Beans 244
Bean Spread 246
Beans Soaking Time 244
Beverages 142
Breakfast Chia 29
Butternut Squash Soup 238
Cardamom Almond Cookies .. 258
"Caesar" Salad 255
Chocolate Chia 'Pudding' 259
Chocolate Chip Cookies 151
Creamy Asparagus Soup 102
Crock-Pot/Slow Cooker 237
Cumin Avocado Dressing 254
Dijon Mustard 250
Dressing 140
Flavored Water 49
Gingered Black Beans 245
Ginger-Garlic Sauce 252
Golden Milk Recipe 236
Granola Bars 256
Hollandaise Sauce 107
Hot Chocolate 30
Hummus 245
Ice Cream 259
Ketchup 250
'Mayo' Dressing 251
Millet "Mashed Potatoes" 242
Miso - Sesame Butter Dip 254

"Morning Apple Pie" 134
Morning Rice 232
Mustard 250
Nut Milk 234
Nut Milk Variations 235
Overnight Oats 232
Popcorn 90
Protein Shakes 134
Quinoa Bean Burgers 241
Quinoa Tabouli 243
Recipe Alterations 150
Rice Drink 'Horchata' 235
Root Soup 239
Sauerkraut 124
Seed Cheeze 247
Simple Grain Free Pancakes 231
Simple Guacamole 249
Slow Cooked Grains 237
S'mores 83
Steel Cut Oatmeal 233
Stevia 85
Sweet Carrot Butter 248
Sweet Potato Chips 261
Sweet Potato Pie 260
Tahini Dressing 196
Tangy Rice Pilaf 240
The Crock Pot / Nuts 237
Trail Mix 257
Vegan Cashew Cream Frosting 258
Vegan Cashew Ranch Dressing 253
Vegan Cheeze 246
Vegan Egg Substitute 231
Vegan 'Hollandaise' Sauce 249
Vegan 'Mayo' 251
Vegan Sour Cream 248
Vegan Sweet Cream 260
Veggie Pizza 243
Worcestershire-ish Sauce 107
Zucchini Pasta 242

Additional Resources

Add-Ins/Upgrades 28
Beverage Upgrades 142
Breakfast Options 158
Blood Sugar Stabilization 114
Create your own Dressing 140
Create your own Sauce 108
Condiments 138
Dairy Upgrades 135
Enzymatic Foods 120
How to Grow Sprouts 184
How to Prep Frozen Meals 184
I Can List 182
Index of Healing Foods 164
Ingredient Conversions 152
Kitchen Sanctuary 189
Meal Upgrades 136
My Upgrade List 150
Nourishing Foods 59
Organic Shopping Tips 57
Probiotic Foods 122
Recipe Alterations 150
Refined Sugar Upgrades 154
Snacks 137, 114
UPGRADED Sweeteners 77, 83-85

* Food/Mood Journal 126

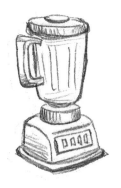

Simple Grain Free Pancakes

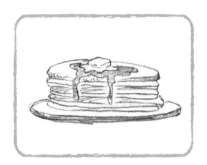

- ❋ 2 pasture raised eggs (or see egg substitute below)
- ❋ 4 oz sweet potato puree (or pumpkin)
- ❋ 1/4 tsp cinnamon
- ❋ 1/4 tsp Celtic Sea Salt
- ❋ 1 TBSP extra virgin coconut oil

Directions:

1. In a warm skillet, add dollop of coconut oil and let it melt to coat the pan.
2. Mix all remaining ingredients together well.
3. Turn stove-top to medium-high heat. Spoon in the batter. The smaller the pancakes, the easier to flip.
4. The heat of your stove-top determines how quickly/slowly the pancakes will cook.
5. Check the bottom of the pancake. When brown, flip over. Cook 2-3 more minutes, remove and serve.
6. Topping options: Coconut Nectar, Chopped bananas and Raw Honey, Maple Syrup, Date or Apricot Syrup (dried fruit syrup: make by soaking dried fruit overnight)

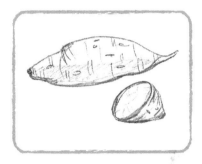

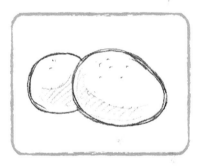

Vegan Egg Substitute

- ❋ 1 TBSP ground flax seeds
- ❋ 2-3 TBSP purified water

Directions:

1. Simmer flax seeds and water in a saucepan for approximately 5 minutes OR until a thick, egg-like consistency.
2. Let this cool before using in a recipe (about 10 minutes).*

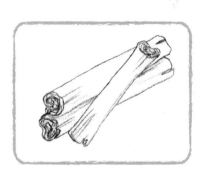

*Note: This recipe makes about 1 egg's worth.

For more, use a ratio of 1 part (flax) to 3 parts (water).
1 cup ground flax seeds and 3 cups water (about 15 eggs worth).
Use about 1/4 cup (about 4 TBSP) flax substitute for every egg needed.

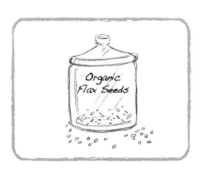

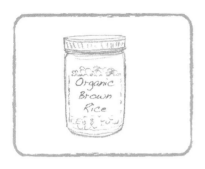

Morning Rice

* 2 cups leftover organic rice (you can use any whole grain)
* ½ tsp cinnamon
* 1 cup purified water
* 2 TBSP toasted sunflower seeds
* Optional: 1 tsp coconut oil

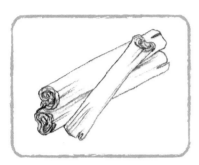

Directions:

1. Bring water and cinnamon to a boil.
2. Place rice in boiling water, cover and simmer for 5 minutes, and then stir.
3. For creamier cereal, mix rice with ½ cup extra water in the blender, then simmer for 15 minutes with cinnamon. Top with toasted seeds.

You can add :
* toasted seeds
* yogurt
* nut milk
* apples
* chopped nuts/seeds
* nut butter
* raisins
* cinnamon etc.

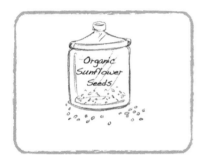

Dry roast cereal for a nuttier flavor before cooking. Oat flakes are especially delicious and heartier when toasted.

Overnight Oats

* ½ cup of whole oat groats
* ½ cup brown rice
* 1 pinch Celtic Sea Salt
* 4 cups of purified water
* 1/4 tsp cinnamon

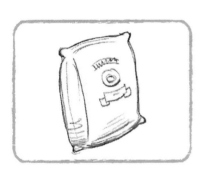

Directions:

1. Place all ingredients in crock pot.
2. Turn heat to high until water boils. Turn to low, cover, and cook overnight.
3. In the morning, open and serve.
4. Add your favorite organic toppings: nuts, seeds, fresh berries, and cinnamon.

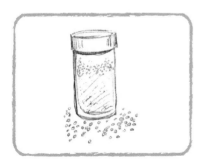

Steel Cut Oatmeal

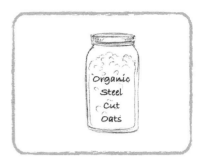

* 1 cup steel-cut oats
* 2 cups purified water
* 2 cups nut milk
* 1/2 cup almond butter
* 3 tablespoons Upgraded Sweetener
  (Coconut Sugar, Raw Honey, Grade B Maple Syrup)
* 1/2 cup goji berries (raisins, dates, fresh
  or dried fruit of your choice)
* 1/4 tsp cinnamon

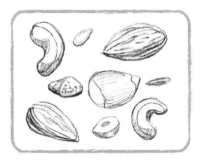

Directions:
1. Soak oats, water and milk.
2. Cover and refrigerate overnight.
3. In saucepan, add almond butter, sweetener, and Goji berries
   and bring to a boil.
4. Lower heat and let it simmer gently.
5. Cook uncovered, stirring frequently until soft
   (approximately 9-12 minutes).

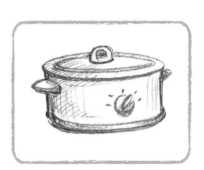

Steel Cut Oats in the Crock Pot

* 1 cup steel-cut oats
* 4 1/2 cups purified water
* 1/4 tsp cinnamon
* 1/2 tsp Celtic Sea Salt
* 2-3 TBSP coconut oil or coconut butter
* 1/2 cup fresh berries
* Stevia or Upgraded Sweetener (to taste)

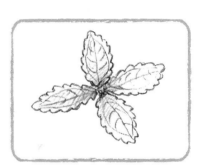

Directions:
1. Place all ingredients in a 2 quart slow cooker.
2. Cover and cook on LOW for 6-8 hours.
3. If a 'crust' forms around the outside, scrape it down
   with a spoon and then stir.

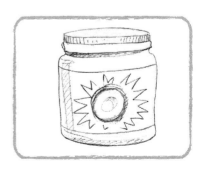

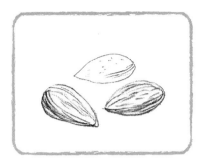

Almond Milk

* ¼ cup almonds
* 1 cup purified water

Directions:

1. In blender, grind almonds into fine flour, and then add water.
2. You can leave it like this or strain through a nut milk bag for a smoother texture.
3. Once the nut milk is at the consistency you desire, add any of the following ingredients:
   * Pinch of Celtic Sea Salt
   * ½ tsp organic cinnamon
   * ½ tsp organic cardamom
   * 2-4 drops of stevia extract or 1/8 tsp (or less) powdered stevia or Upgraded Sweetener of choice (page 83-85).

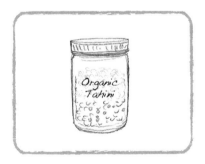

Variations:

* 1/3 cup sunflower seeds **or**
* 1/3 cup pumpkin seeds **or**
* 1/4 cup pecans **or**
* 1/3 cup walnuts, etc.

A simpler option and my favorite way to make Nut Milk:

* 1 TBSP almond butter
* 1 Cup purified water
* 1 dash green stevia powder
* A splash of vanilla extract
* Celtic Sea Salt to taste
* Sprinkle of cinnamon

Play with the ingredient amounts to make it taste good to you.

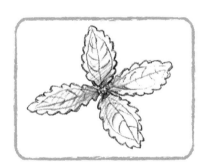

Directions:

1. In a blender, place all ingredients together and blend.
2. Use as is or place in a small saucepan and bring to medium heat, then serve.

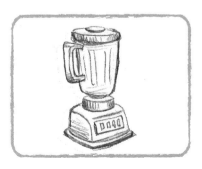

Nut Milk Variations:

* 1 Cup water
* 1 TBSP coconut oil or butter
* 1 TBSP nut/seed butter (Use any nut/seed/coconut butter)

Add-In Options:
* Cinnamon
* Upgraded Sweetener
* Celtic Sea Salt

Nut milk keeps for many days in the fridge.
* Shake before serving.

* Put in your favorite container to take with you.

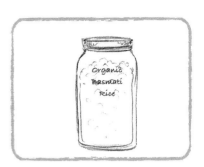

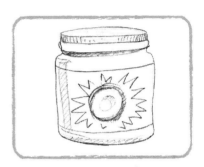

Rice Drink 'Horchata'

* 1 cup cooked brown or basmati rice
* 5 cups water
* ½ cup milk (coconut, hemp, almond or organic grass fed milk)
* 2 tsp vanilla extract
* 2 tsp ground cinnamon
* 1 TBSP maca root
* 2/3 cup coconut sugar
* 1 TBSP coconut oil (optional)

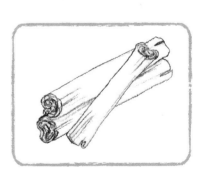

Directions:
1. Make sure the rice is cool to the touch. Place rice and water in a blender.
2. Blend on medium high speed for about 1-2 minutes, or until rice is broken up.
3. Pour into a strainer and remove the rice fiber (leaving just the liquid).
4. Stir in milk, vanilla, cinnamon, maca, and coconut sugar into rice liquid.
5. Serve warm or cold. When serving warm, place ingredients in a sauce pan, add coconut oil, and bring to medium heat.
6. Stir mixture occasionally and turn off the heat before mixture comes to a boil. Cool and then pour into your favorite mug.

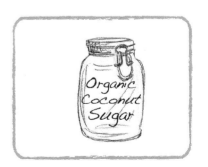

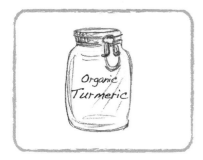

Golden Milk Recipe
(Sleep, hormones and pain tonic)

Ingredients:

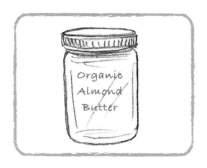

* 1/2 - 2 tsp turmeric powder (start with 1/2 tsp and slowly increase to desired amount)
* 1 cup of almond milk or any milk (unsweetened) OR - 1 TBSP almond butter & 1 cup purified water
* 1 tsp extra virgin coconut oil
* 1/4 tsp cardamom
* 1/4 tsp of cinnamon (optional)
* 1 tsp *maca root powder (optional)

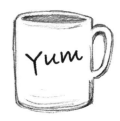

Directions:

1. Over medium heat, pour the turmeric, almond milk, and spices into pan until WARM.
2. Add sweetener of your choices: dash of green leaf stevia, grade B maple syrup or coconut sugar OR drizzle of raw honey.
3. Pour into a favorite mug and enjoy!

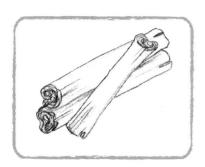

*Maca root is a medicinal plant that grows in Peru. It's a relative of the radish and has a butterscotch aroma. It helps increase fertility in livestock and women, and is a hormone balancer for men. It can also assist with female hormonal balance (a client raves that it reduced her hot flashes when nothing else worked). It can help improve anemia, memory, depression, menstrual problems, osteoporosis, stomach issues, sexual problems, and helps boost the immune system.

Maca Root powder can be used in drinks, smoothies, and baked into food. My favorite is to add it to raw chocolate and can also be used in soups. Look for organic gelatinized Maca (sometimes easier to digest than raw Maca). When purchasing Maca, make sure that it's the ONLY ingredient.

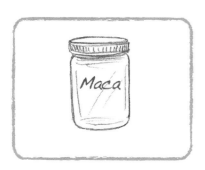

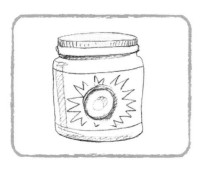

Crock-Pot/Slow Cooker

The crock-pot is an excellent kitchen tool. Experiment with one pot meals on the stove top or in the crock-pot for easy, delicious, nutritious slow cooked meals. Experiment with making a simple vegetable soup and slow cook all day until you are ready for dinner.

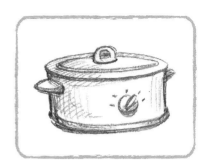

If you like, experiment with slow cooking your breakfast so that it's ready for you in the morning.

The Crock Pot Has Gone Nuts!

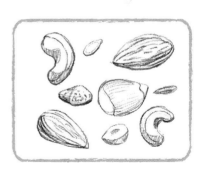

* 24 oz unsalted raw or dry-roasted organic cashews, almonds, pecans, walnuts, sunflower seeds
  and/or pumpkin seeds
* 1/4 cup organic extra virgin coconut oil
* Cajun seasoning mix (or any favorite natural organic seasonings)

Directions:
1. Mix nuts/seeds oil and seasoning well.
2. Place in crock pot on low for 2 hours. Stir and check occasionally.
3. Remove lid.
4. Turn heat to high and cook for about 10 minutes.
5. Eat warm or put into nut dishes.

Slow Cooked Grains
* All grains can be slow cooked as well.

Directions:
1. Place water, grain, seaweed, and sea salt into a crock pot or slow cooker.
2. Turn on high until boiling. Skim off any foam.
3. Turn to low, cover, and cook 6-8 hours.

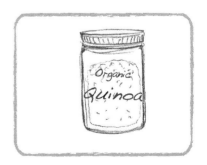

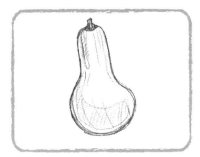

Slow Cooked Butternut Squash Soup

* 1 medium yellow onion, chopped
* 3 medium carrots, chopped
* 3 medium celery stalks, chopped
* 1 medium butternut squash, chopped
  (remove the skin and seeds)
* 1 large apple, peeled and chopped
  (use your favorite kind of apple, I usually use a Granny
  Smith or Fuji)
* 1 TBSP coconut oil
* 1/2 tsp cinnamon
* 1/4 tsp nutmeg
* Celtic Sea Salt and ground pepper to taste

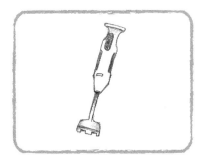

Directions:

1. Add ingredients to the slow cooker.
2. Cook on low for 6-8 hours or on high for 3-4 hours.
3. When vegetables are soft, use a metal hand held blender.
4. Once you've blended the vegetables, you can add spice to your
   liking and keep in the crock pot until you are ready to serve.

If you don't have a hand held metal immersion blender:
1. Turn off heat and wait for the vegetables to cool.
2. Transfer to a blender and blend.
   OR Mash and eat chunky-style.

*Never put hot liquids into blender, because it could expand and
go everywhere (not fun).

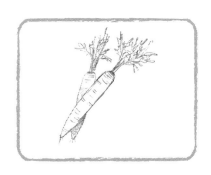

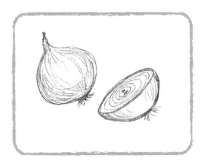

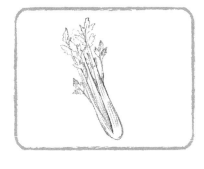

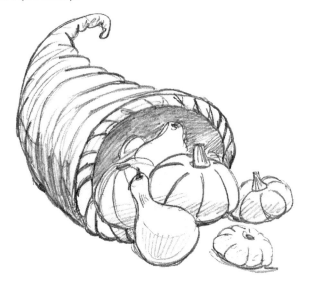

Root Soup

* 4 organic sweet potatoes, peeled and diced
* 1 organic onion, chopped
* 1 organic garlic clove, cut in half
* 1 organic parsnip, peeled and diced
* 2 organic carrots, peeled and diced
* 1 organic turnip, peeled and diced
* 1 organic celery root, peeled and diced (optional)
* 1 organic fennel bulb, diced (optional)
* 1 organic leek, washed and thinly sliced
* 1 organic rutabaga, peeled and diced
* 4 cups organic vegetable broth
* 1/3 cup organic brown rice or basmati rice
* 1/3 cup organic cilantro, washed and chopped
* 4 cups purified water
* Celtic Sea Salt and pepper to taste

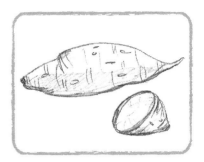

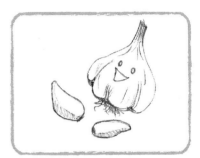

Directions:

1. Pre-cook brown or basmati rice.
2. If using quinoa, add in last 20 minutes of cooking.
3. Add remaining ingredients to a large sauce pan and bring to a boil.
4. Simmer until all of the vegetables are tender (about 40 minutes uncovered).
5. If needed, add more water.
6. When tender, serve as is or use a potato masher or immersion blender until desired consistency.

   * Never put hot liquids into a blender.

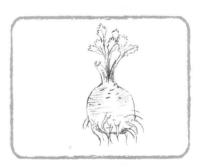

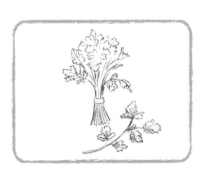

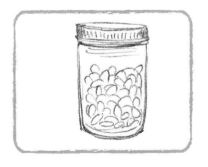

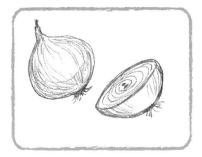

Basic Vegetable Broth

- ❋ 1 TBSP extra virgin coconut oil
- ❋ 2 medium white, red or yellow onions, peeled and chopped
- ❋ 3 medium carrots, cut into 1-inch pieces
- ❋ 2 celery stalks, cut into 1-inch pieces
- ❋ 3-4 garlic cloves, peeled
- ❋ 3/4 cup parsley, chopped
- ❋ 1 bay leaf
- ❋ 1 tsp Celtic Sea Salt
- ❋ 8 cups purified water

Directions:

1. In large stock pot, put the coconut oil in first and allow it to melt.
2. Add the rest of the ingredients, stir and cover.
3. Cook on low for 8-10 hours.
4. Turn off and allow broth to cool.
5. Once cool, you can strain it through a fine mesh into another pot.
6. Push with a wooden spoon to get out remaining juices.
7. Store in glass jars. Keep for 3-5 days in the fridge, or freeze portions for later use.

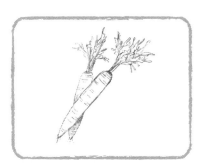

When freezing glass jars, make sure you use ones that don't have 'shoulders'. Use the straight jars for freezing to avoid cracking that can happen with expansion in the freezer. When freezing glass jars, make sure to leave at least an inch from the top to avoid the jar from cracking. Note: most store bought broths are full of table salt and often MSG and other undesirables.

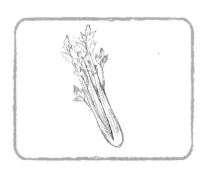

Tangy Rice Pilaf

- ❋ 2 cups basmati rice
- ❋ ½ onion, sliced
- ❋ 1 cup cabbage, diced
- ❋ 1 uemboshi plum, pitted
- ❋ ¾ cup purified water

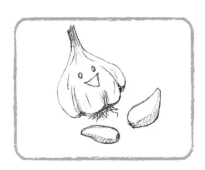

Directions:

1. Mince the uemboshi plum.
2. Spread the uemboshi plum in a skillet and add vegetables.
3. Lay the rice on top and add water. Bring to a boil.
4. Cover, lower heat, and simmer for 5-8 minutes or until the cabbage is tender.
5. Toss and serve.

- ❋ Uemboshi plum is a digestive aid and has a tangy flavor.

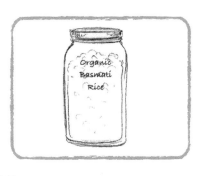

Quinoa Bean Burgers

- ❋ 2 cups cooked beans
- ❋ 1 carrot, diced
- ❋ 1/4 onion, diced (optional)
- ❋ 1/4 cup fresh cilantro and/or parsley
- ❋ 1/2 cup quinoa or amaranth
- ❋ Celtic Sea Salt to taste
- ❋ Toasted nuts or seeds

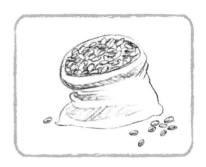

Directions:

1. Mash beans.
2. Mix ingredients together and form patties or small balls.
3. On a baking sheet, spread a little bit of coconut oil.
4. Bake at 350 degrees until browned.

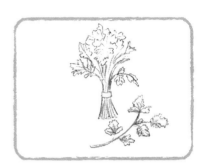

Baked Amaranth Veggie Patties

- ❋ 1 cup organic amaranth
- ❋ 2 cups purified water
- ❋ 1 TBSP organic coconut or olive oil
- ❋ 3 cups organic spinach
- ❋ 2 organic carrots – grated
- ❋ ¼ cup nutritional yeast
  or grass fed cheese or sheep/goat cheese
- ❋ ½ tsp baking powder
- ❋ 3 TBSP almond butter
- ❋ 1 handful fresh basil
- ❋ ½ juiced lime
- ❋ 1 tsp Celtic Sea Salt

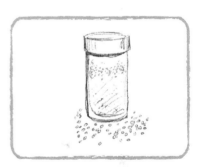

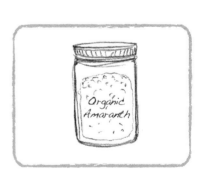

Directions:

1. Preheat oven to 400 degrees. Line a baking sheet with parchment paper and then lightly oil.
2. Place amaranth and water in pot and bring to a boil. Cover and simmer for 20 minutes until amaranth is soft and water is absorbed. Remove lid and fluff. Set aside to cool.
3. Add carrots and spinach and cook until wilted.
4. In a large mixing bowl, mix amaranth, cooked veggies, and all remaining ingredients. Mix with hands until it is all uniformly combined.
5. Taste and adjust seasonings to taste. Shape and make about 10 patties.
6. Bake 20-30 minutes until golden and crunchy on top. Serve as is or topped with a dab of your favorite sauce.

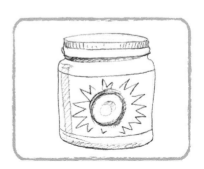

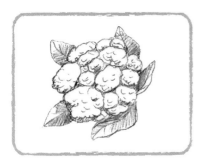

Millet "Mashed Potatoes"

* 1 cup millet
* 2 ¼ cups purified water
* ½ medium cauliflower
* 1 TBSP coconut oil
* 1 TBSP organic, raw apple cider vinegar
* 1/4 tsp Celtic Sea Salt

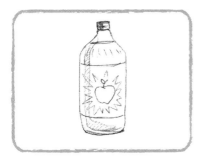

Directions:

1. Wash grains. Bring water to a boil, and add grains, cauliflower and garlic.
2. Reduce heat to low and simmer covered for 20 minutes or until grains are cooked.
   and water is absorbed.
3. Turn off heat, and let sit covered for 5-10 minutes
4. Add other ingredients and mash with a potato masher, or mix in a blender or food processor.
5. Garnish and serve.
6. For a slightly "cheesy" texture add a few tablespoons of nutritional yeast.
7. You can garnish with chopped organic parsley or favorite organic garnish, and spice according to taste.
8. You can also add roasted garlic and onion.

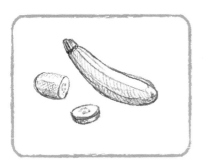

Zucchini Pasta

* 2 zucchinis
* ½ cup extra virgin olive oil
* ¼ tsp black pepper
* 2 garlic cloves (finely cut)

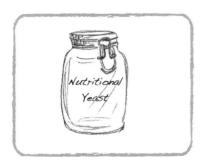

Directions:

1. Chop zucchini into matchsticks or push through a spiralizer machine.
2. In a blender place olive oil, pepper and garlic.
3. Blend until smooth.
4. Pour on top of zucchini!

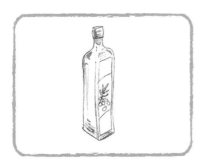

Veggie Pizza

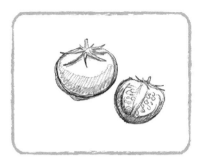

* Sprouted grain pizza crust
* 7 oz glass jar of organic tomato paste
  (in glass jar/no sugar)
* 16 oz glass jar of organic tomato or pizza/pasta sauce
  (check ingredients, find one without sugar)
* 1 bunch of fresh basil
* 1 tsp garlic powder
* 1/2 cup shiitake mushrooms
* 1 small orange bell pepper
* Vegan Cheezy sauce (see recipe) OR Grass Fed Cheese

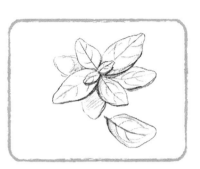

Directions:

1. Mix together the pizza sauce and tomato paste to make a thick sauce.
2. With a spatula, spread combined sauce evenly over the pizza crust.
3. Dust lightly with a layer of the garlic powder.
4. Gently pour ¾ of the cheesy sauce over pizza (so you don't mix it with the pizza sauce).
5. Top with shiitake mushrooms, orange bell peppers, and fresh herbs.
6. Bake at 425 degrees for 15 minutes or until crust is brown and crisp.

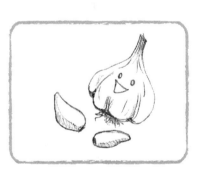

Quinoa Tabouli

* 1 cup quinoa
* 2 cups purified water
* 1 cup parsley, chopped
* 1/4 onion, diced (optional)
* 1 tomato, diced
* Juice of 1 lemon (freshly squeezed)
* 1 tsp coconut oil or olive oil
* 1/2 tsp Celtic Sea Salt
* 2 tbs fresh organic mint, chopped or
* 1 tsp dried organic mint

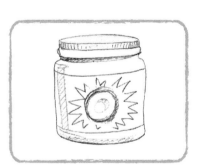

Directions:

1. Mix all ingredients together.
2. Garnish with cilantro and parsley.

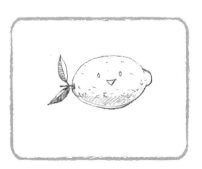

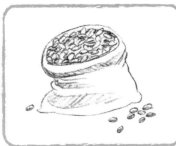

Beans

When selecting protein sources, beans are a great choice! They are packed with iron, B vitamins, and fiber.

How to Prepare Dry Beans

1. Pick through your beans to remove any rocks or withered beans.
2. Rinse beans in cool water. Place the beans in a container and cover with water that covers them four inches higher than the beans.
3. After soaking for six hours, drain and rinse the beans again.
4. Put the beans in a heavy pot with 3-4 cups of water. Bring the water to a boil making sure to remove the foam as it appears.
5. To add flavor to the beans, you can add kombu, bay leaves, or garlic. This will also help make the beans easier to digest.
6. Cover the pot and simmer for the time suggested. If the beans are soft in the middle, they are done!
7. During the last ten minutes, add some Celtic Sea Salt for flavoring.

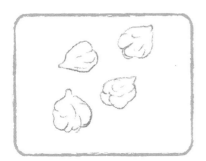

Digesting Beans and Avoiding Gas

Some people struggle to eat beans and legumes because they are hard to digest. Some ways to make them easier to digest: allow them to soak for several days, use a pressure cooker, and chew beans thoroughly. You may also wish to try different types of beans. Adzuki, lentils, mung beans, and peas are the easiest to digest. This can also be helped by adding apple cider vinegar.

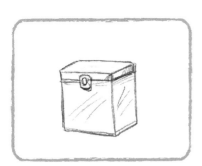

Beans Soaking Time:

1 cup dry beans	Cooking time
✽ adzuki	45-60 minutes
✽ anasazi	60-90 minutes
✽ black (turtle)	60-90 minutes
✽ black-eyed peas	60 minutes
✽ cannellini	90-120 minutes
✽ chickpeas (garbanzos)	120-180 minutes
✽ fava	60-90 minutes
✽ great northern	90-120 minutes
✽ kidney	60-90 minutes
✽ Lentils	30-45 minutes
✽ lima beans	60-90 minutes
✽ mung	60 minutes
✽ navy	60-90 minutes
✽ pinto	90 minutes
✽ split peas	45-60 minutes

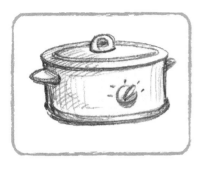

Gingered Black Beans

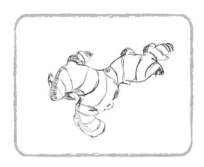

* 1½ cup black turtle beans
* 4 cups purified water
* 1 strip kombu seaweed
* 2 tsp coconut aminos
* 1 tsp finely grated ginger

Directions:

1. Sort beans, wash, and soak overnight.
2. Place in pot and boil uncovered for 5 minutes.
3. Skim off the foam (this reduces gas).
4. Add kombu, cover, and bring to a boil.
5. Turn down heat and cook for 2-3 hours.
6. Add ginger and simmer for another 10 minutes.
7. Turn off heat, add in coconut aminos, and stir.

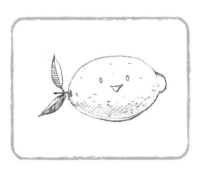

Hummus

* 2 cups cooked organic garbanzo beans
* 1/4 cup ground organic sesame seeds
  or 1/4 cup organic tahini
* 1-3 cloves of organic garlic, minced
* 6-8 TBSP of organic lemon juice (fresh squeezed)
* Dash of organic cayenne pepper
* 1 TBSP of organic olive oil (optional)
* Celtic Sea Salt to taste

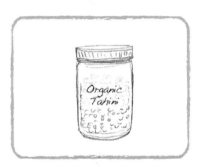

Directions:

1. Mash or puree garbanzo beans with the rest of the ingredients.
2. Spread on plate and garnish with parsley and cilantro.
3. Serve as a dip with carrots, celery, jicama, etc.

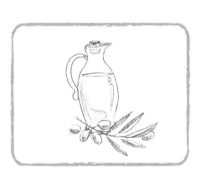

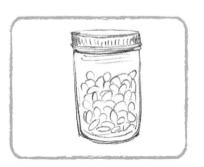

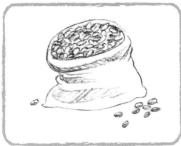

Bean Spread

* 2 cups lentils, kidney, black, pinto **or** garbanzo beans
* 1 stalk celery, minced fine
* 1 green onion, sliced
* 2 TBSP minced parsley
* 2 TBSP minced cilantro
* 2 TBSP lemon juice (fresh squeezed)
* 2 tsp chickpea miso
* ¼ cup ground roasted sunflower or
* sesame seeds to taste

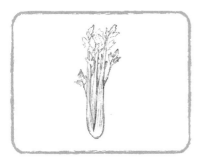

Directions:

1. Toast the seeds by stirring in a skillet over medium heat until they smell and taste nutty (not too browned or they will have a bitter taste).

2. Grind seeds in a blender until powdered. Mash the beans with a potato masher or fork.

3. Mix all the ingredients and add seasoning to taste.

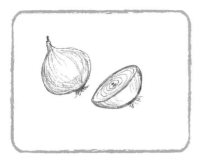

Vegan Cheeze

* 2/3 cup purified water
* 1 1/4 cup almonds or pecans
* 3 TBSP lemon juice (fresh squeezed)
* 1/4 cup nutritional yeast
* 1/4 cup red bell pepper
* 1 tsp paprika
* 1 tsp Celtic Sea Salt
* 1/8 tsp cayenne pepper

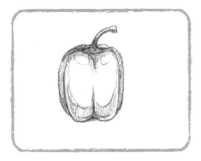

Directions:

1. Place all ingredients into the blender and pulse a few times.

2. Blend until desired consistency.

3. For a thicker sauce, use less water. For a thinner sauce, use more water.

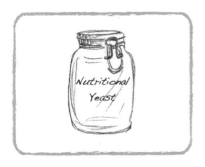

Seed Cheeze

- 1 cup raw sunflower seeds
- 1/2 cup raw brown sesame seeds
- ½ tsp Celtic Sea Salt or Himalayan salt
- 24-32 oz ball jar with sprouting lid
- 7 cups purified water
  (4 cups for soaking and approx. 3 cups for blending)

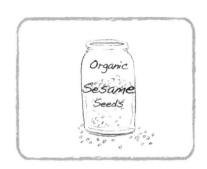

Directions:

1. Place sunflower seeds and sesame seeds in a glass jar. Make sure that the amount of the seeds fill only half of the jar (they need room to expand).

2. Add at least 4 cups of purified water to fully immerse seeds (seeds will expand). Do not fill water to the top. Leave at least 1-2" from the top of the jar.

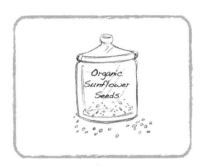

3. Place sprouting lid on jar and soak for 8 hours.

4. After seeds have soaked for 8 hours (if you have a sprouting lid on the jar that is secure), turn the jar upside down and drain water. If you have a rack, leave the jar upside down, so water drains out or get as much water out as you can. Place on the counter-top.

5. After sitting for another 8 hours (this is the sprouting time), add seeds to a food processor or blend on low speed. Add Celtic Sea Salt or Himalayan Salt.

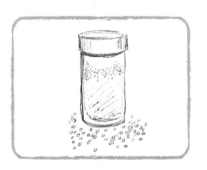

6. Have 3 cups purified water handy and SLOWLY add in liquid as you blend. Start with 1 cup and then add as needed. You may need more water or you may need less. Look for a consistency that isn't too dry but not too wet either.

7. Once you reach a desired consistency, place blended mixture into large ball jar.

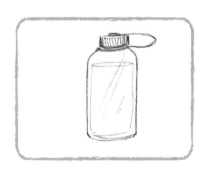

8. Put sprout lid back on or cover with a dishcloth. Keep jar in a dark, cool place for 8 hours.

9. The seed cheese will EXPAND so make sure the jar has at least 4-5 inches of room at the top. If you only have small jars, portion into two or three separate jars. Leave room at top for expansion.

10. After 8 hours, your seed cheese is ready to eat. Store in fridge for 2-3 days. Sometimes the cheese lasts longer and sometimes it doesn't.

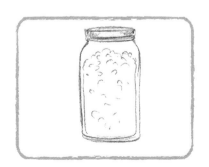

11. If you want the seed cheeze to taste more sour, experiment with longer fermentation times.

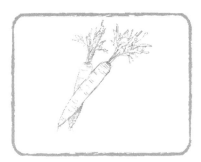

Sweet Carrot Butter

* 4 cups carrots, sliced
* ½ cup purified water
* Pinch of Celtic Sea Salt
* 1 heaping TBSP of kuzu dissolved in 2 TBSP of purified water
* 1-2 TBSP of organic sesame tahini

Directions:

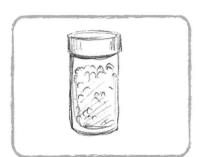

1. Slice carrots and place in pressure cooker with water and salt.
2. Bring to pressure, turn down and simmer 10 minutes.
   * If you don't have a pressure cooker, steam 20 minutes.
3. Puree carrots in blender with ½ cup liquid from pressure cooking or steaming.
4. Dissolve kuzu in cool water, mix with carrot puree, and reheat.
5. Stir until it bubbles (kuzu must be heated thoroughly to thicken).
6. For buttery flavor, stir in sesame tahini. SO Delicious!

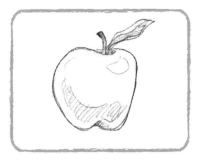

Apple Butter

* 11 organic apples
* 1/2 cup purified water
* 2 tsp cinnamon
* Add stevia or natural sweetener to taste (optional)

Directions:

1. Wash and peel apples. Cut into quarters, remove seeds.
2. Combine water & cinnamon then pour into crock pot over apples.
3. Cook on low all day.
4. For a creamy texture, let cool and then blend to desired consistency. YUM!

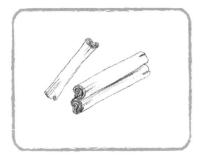

Vegan Sour Cream

* 2 cups almonds, soaked
* 2 TBSP lemon juice (freshly squeezed)
* 1 clove garlic, minced

Directions:

1. Place all ingredients into the blender and pulse a few times.
2. Blend until desired consistency.

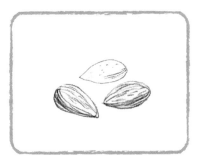

Simple Guacamole

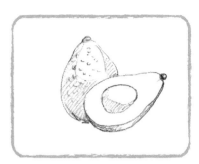

- ✱ 1 medium or large avocado
- ✱ 1/4 tomato, diced
- ✱ 1 clove garlic, minced
- ✱ 1 tsp onion, minced
- ✱ dash of cayenne pepper
- ✱ 1-3 tsp of lime juice (fresh squeezed)
- ✱ 1/3 cilantro, chopped
- ✱ Celtic sea salt to taste

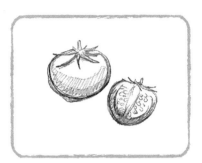

Directions:
1. Combine and mash with a fork.
2. For a smoother guacamole, put into a blender and 'pulse' until desired consistency.

Vegan 'Hollandaise' Sauce

- ✱ ¾ cup coconut oil
- ✱ ½ cup walnuts
- ✱ ¼ cup lemon juice (fresh squeezed)
- ✱ 1 avocado
- ✱ 1 TBSP nutritional yeast
- ✱ 1 tsp Celtic Sea Salt
- ✱ ¼ tsp cayenne
- ✱ ¼ tsp turmeric

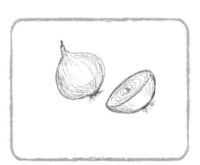

Directions:
1. Place all ingredients into a blender and blend until desired consistency.
2. Add a little water or a bit more lemon juice if too thick.

Delicious when poured over freshly steamed organic asparagus!

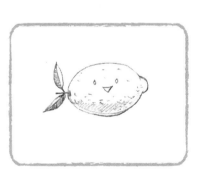

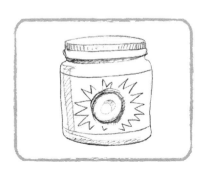

Ketchup

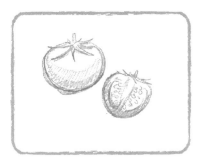

* 1 cup sun-dried tomatoes (soaked in purified water)
* 1 cup tomatoes, diced
* 1 cup purified water (save soak water from tomatoes)
* 2 TBSP raw organic apple cider vinegar
* 1/2 tsp Celtic sea salt

Directions:

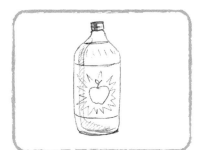

1. Soak sun-dried tomatoes in purified water for about an hour or until soft.
2. Place all ingredients into the blender.
3. Blend until creamy.
4. For a thicker sauce, use less water.
5. For a thinner sauce, use more water.

Mustard

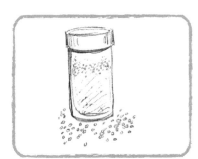

* 2 cups yellow mustard seeds, soaked for 6-8 hours
* 1 cup organic raw apple cider vinegar
* 1 cup purified water
* 1 tsp Celtic Sea Salt

Directions:

1. Place all ingredients into the blender.
2. Blend until creamy.
3. For a thicker sauce, use less water.
4. For a thinner sauce, use more water.

Dijon Mustard

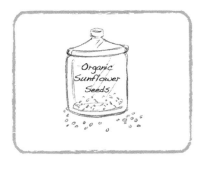

* 3/4 cups sunflower seeds, soaked
* 1/2 cup macadamia nuts
* 3/4 cup purified water
* 1 1/2 TBSP organic apple cider vinegar
* 1 tsp paprika
* 1 tsp mustard powder
* 1 1/2 tsp Celtic sea salt

Directions:

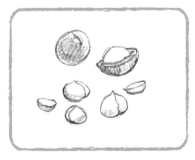

1. Place all ingredients into the blender.
2. Blend until creamy.

Vegan 'Mayo'

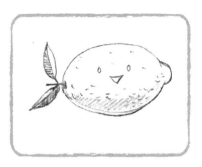

* 1 cup purified water
* 1/4 cup macadamia nuts
* 1/4 cup pine nuts
* 1 TBSP lemon juice (fresh squeezed)
* 1/4 cup olive oil or coconut oil
* 1/4 tsp Celtic Sea Salt
* 1/4 tsp paprika
* 1 clove garlic or 1/8 tsp garlic powder
* 1/4 tsp mustard powder
* 1/8 (or less) tsp of stevia for a hint of sweetness

Directions:

1. Blend all ingredients together until desired consistency.
2. To add a little sweetness, add a pinch to 1/8 tsp of organic green leaf stevia, or a couple drops of liquid stevia.
3. If your blood sugar is stable, add ½-1 TBSP of organic RAW honey.

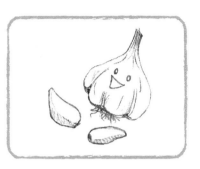

'Mayo' Dressing

* 1 cup of 'Mayo' (above)
* 1/2 tsp garlic powder
* 1/2 tsp onion powder
* 1/4 tsp black pepper
* 2 tsp parsley, chopped
* 1/2 cup unsweetened full fat organic coconut milk
* Celtic sea salt to taste (optional)

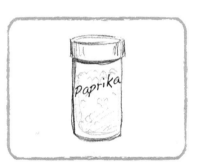

Directions:

1. Place all ingredients into the blender.
2. Blend until creamy.

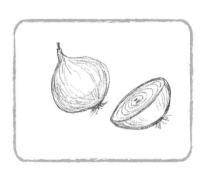

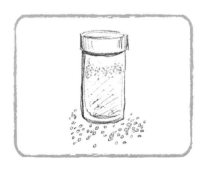

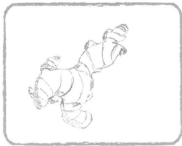

Ginger-Garlic Sauce

* 1/8 cup garlic cloves, peeled
* 1/8 cup ginger root, peeled
* 1/2 cup purified water
* 1/4 TBSP raw honey
* 1/4 tsp pepper
* 1 tsp lemon juice (fresh squeezed)
* 1 cup extra virgin olive oil
* 1/2 cup organic raw apple cider vinegar
* 1/2 cup walnuts

Directions:
1. Place all ingredients in blender.
2. Blend until smooth.
3. Will keep for 1-2 weeks.

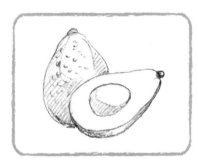

Avocado Mushroom Sauce

* 1TBSP chickpea miso
* 1-2 cloves of organic garlic
* 1/2 " of ginger
* 1" of turmeric
* Juice of ½ lime (fresh squeezed)
* 1 TBSP coconut oil
* 1/4 bunch of cilantro
* 2 TBSP nutritional yeast
* Pinch of Celtic Sea Salt
* Pinch of Cayenne
* 1/2 - 1 avocado
* 1/2 - 1 cup of purified water

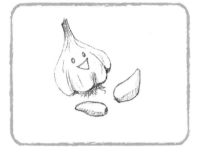

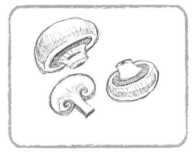

Directions:
1. Place all ingredients in blender.
2. Blend until smooth.
3. Pour over steamed asparagus or vegetable of your choice, Yum!

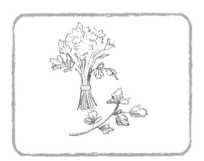

Vegan Cashew Ranch Dressing

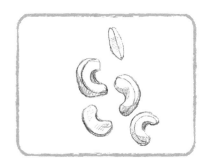

* 1 cup raw cashews
* ¼ cup lemon juice (freshly squeezed)
* ¼ cup organic raw apple cider vinegar
* 2 dates (medjool)
* ½ cup of the water from soaking the dates
* 2-4 cloves of organic garlic
* 1/8 cup chopped onion
* 1-2 tsp Celtic Sea Salt
* 1 TBSP fresh parsley, chopped
* ½ tsp fresh dill, chopped
* 1 TBSP green onions, chopped

Directions:

1. Soak the cashews in purified water for 2 hours. Drain water.
2. Soak the dates in purified water for a few hours before using (optional).
3. Blend ingredients (except for herbs) until creamy and smooth. Add the herbs and stir.
4. When using as a dip, place in the refrigerator to thicken.
5. For dressing, add ½-1 cup water to the blender and blend until desired dressing consistency. Enjoy!

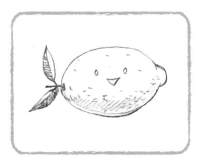

Avocado Lemon Dill Dressing

* 1 medium or large avocado
* 1/2 lemon (juiced)
* 1/2 cup purified water or broth
* 1/2 tsp dill
* 1/4 tsp Celtic Sea Salt

Directions:

1. Place all ingredients in a blender.
2. Blend until smooth.

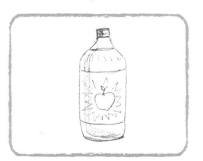

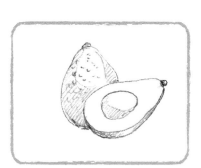

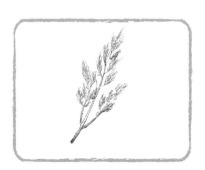

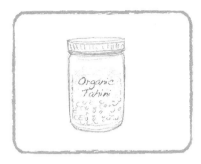

Tahini Dressing

* 1 cup tahini
* 1/2 cup lemon juice (fresh squeezed)
* 1 garlic clove
* Purified water
* Celtic Sea Salt and pepper to taste

Directions:

1. Place all ingredients in blender.
2. Blend until smooth.

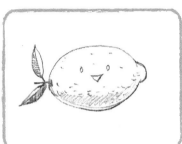

Cumin Avocado Dressing

* 1 tsp ground cumin seeds
* 3 TBSP lime juice (freshly squeezed)
* 3 TBSP extra virgin olive oil
* 1 avocado
* 1/2 tsp Dijon mustard
* 1 garlic clove, minced
* 1/4 cup purified water
* 1/2 tsp Celtic Sea Salt
* Black pepper to taste

Directions:

1. Place all ingredients in blender (except black pepper).
2. Blend until smooth.
3. Slowly add in more water until desired consistency.
4. Add a pinch of black pepper to taste.

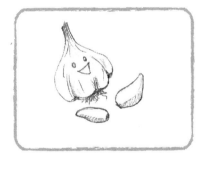

Miso - Sesame Butter Dip

* 1 TBSP chickpea miso
* 1 TBSP sesame butter
* 1/4 cup lemon juice (fresh squeezed)
* 1/4 cup purified water

Directions:

1. Place all ingredients in blender.
2. Blend until smooth.
3. Slowly add in about 1/4 cup water to make this a sauce instead of a dip.

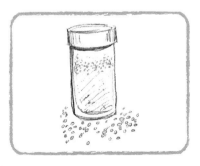

Avocado & Kale Salad

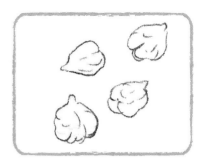

* 1 bunch kale (shredded)
* 1 cup red or orange bell peppers
* 1 medium ripe avocado
* 2 1/2 TBSP olive oil
* 1 2/3 TBSP lemon juice (fresh squeezed)
* 1/4 cup cilantro, chopped
* 1 tsp Celtic Sea Salt (to taste)
* Sprinkle of cayenne pepper to taste (optional)

Directions:

1. Place kale, lemon juice, cilantro and sea salt in a large bowl.
2. Start to 'massage' and 'squeeze' the salad together.
   The sea salt will help to soften the kale.
3. Massage until kale is soft.
4. Add in the rest of the ingredients.
5. Toss and serve.

Add any additional ingredients to your salad.

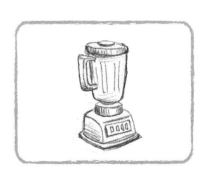

"Caesar" Salad

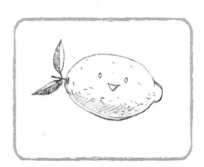

* 1 head of lettuce or bowl of mixed greens (shredded)
* 1 cup 'mayo' (see page 251)
* 1 1/2 tsp mustard or dijon mustard (see page 250)
* 1 clove garlic
* 1 TBSP purified water
* 1 1/2 tsp lemon juice (fresh squeezed)
* 1 1/2 tsp nutritional yeast
* Celtic Sea Salt to taste
* Pepper to taste

Directions:

1. Place all ingredients into a large bowl.
2. Mix together and serve.

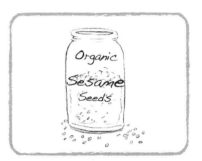

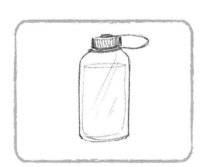

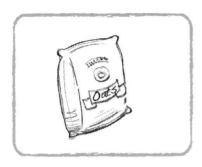

Granola Bars I

* 2-1/2 cups quick rolled oats
* 1 cup raw pumpkin seeds
* 1/2 cup raisins or currants
* 2/3 cup almond butter
* 3/4 cup Upgraded Sweetener (see below)
* 1/8 tsp cinnamon
* Celtic Sea Salt to taste

Nuts/seeds:

Use any kind of nut or seed you prefer, some options:

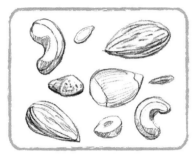

* Sunflower Seeds
* Flax Seeds
* Brazil Nuts
* Hazelnuts
* Pine Nuts

* Sesame Seeds
* Almonds
* Cashews
* Pecans
* Walnuts

Get creative with your snacks!

Sweetener options (pages 77, 83-85):

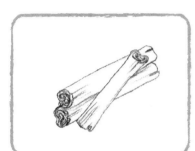

* Brown Rice Syrup
* Grade B Maple Syrup
* Coconut Nectar

Directions:

1. Mix the oats, pumpkin seeds, and currants together.
2. Mix the nut butter, sweetener (start with 1/2 cup - add more if they don't stick together well), cinnamon, and sea salt.
3. Add oats and mix well until everything is sticky. If it's too dry, add a little more sweetener.
4. Line a shallow baking dish with plastic wrap. Press mixture into dish.
5. Place in refrigerator for 3-4 hours. Cut into bars of desired shape, wrap individually, and keep in the refrigerator until ready to eat.

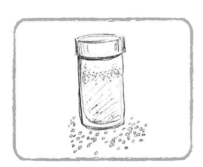

*Note: The almond butter mixed with the Brown Rice Syrup or Organic Grade B Maple Syrup will help stick the ingredients together. While this is a high glycemic snack, I promise you that it's healthier than most of the granola bars on the market. Enjoy!

Granola Bars II

* 1-1/2 cups chopped raw or dry roasted almonds
* 1-1/2 cups raw or dry roasted chopped cashews
* 1 cup shredded, unsweetened coconut
* 1-1/2 cups sunflower and/or pumpkin seeds
* 3 TBSP coconut oil, melted
* 3/4 cups raw honey, grade B maple syrup,
* Brown rice syrup OR coconut nectar
* 1 TBSP vanilla powder or extract
* 1/4 tsp Celtic Sea Salt

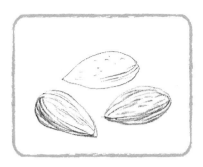

Directions:

1. Preheat oven to 300 degrees. Line an 11" x 7" (approx.) baking pan with coconut oil or parchment paper.
2. Mix together almonds, cashews, seeds, and shredded coconut.
3. Place coconut oil, sweetener and sea salt in a small pan and heat on low until it melts.
4. Add vanilla powder or extract to the nut/seed/coconut mixture and mix well.
5. Line dish with parchment paper. Pour the mixture into pan and press into the bottom.
6. Bake for 30 minutes. COOL completely BEFORE cutting (otherwise they will fall apart). You can also place in refrigerator for approximately 2 hours before cutting as well.
7. Once cool, remove from baking dish and cut into desired size.
8. Store in airtight container or bags.
   These granola bars will keep for about a week.

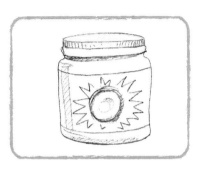

Trail Mix

* 1 cup goji berries (raisins, currants, dates etc.)
* 1 cup sunflower seeds
* 1 cup almonds
* 1 cup cacao nibs
* 1 tsp Celtic Sea Salt (to taste)

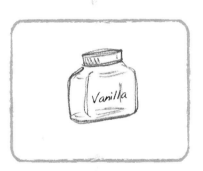

Directions:

1. Combine in a container, shake shake shake senora!
2. Divide trail mix and place in individual baggies!
3. Store in the refrigerator and grab two baggies on your way out the door!

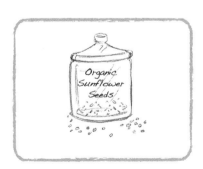

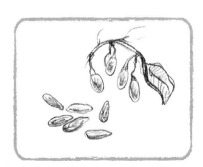

257

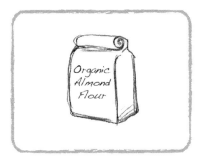

Cardamom Almond Cookies

* 1 cup raw almonds
* 1/4 cup, grade B maple syrup
* 1/8 - 1/4 tsp ground cardamom
* 1/8 - 1/4 tsp ground cinnamon
* 1/8 tsp ground vanilla (optional) or 2-3 drops of vanilla extract
* 2 TBSP purified water
* Coconut oil (for greased baking sheet)

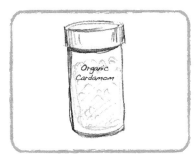

Directions:

1. Preheat oven to 300 degrees.
2. Finely grind almonds in a food processor or blender.
3. Mix in the cardamom, cinnamon, vanilla, maple syrup and water.
4. Create drop balls of the dough and place on a well oiled (coconut oil) cookie sheet.
5. Bake for 15-20 minutes or until lightly golden brown. Let cool, and remove with a spatula and enjoy!

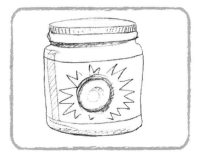

Vegan Cashew Cream Frosting

* 2 cups raw cashews (soak 1 hour)
* 1-2 TBSP lemon juice (fresh squeezed)
* 2 TBSP extra virgin coconut oil
* stevia to taste (or if you can't do stevia, 1/3 cup organic grade B maple syrup)
* Purified water, as needed

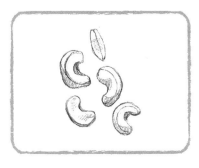

Directions

1. Blend soaked cashews, lemon juice, and coconut oil in a blender until smooth.
2. Add just a little bit of water at a time until desired consistency. Add stevia to taste.
3. Place in refrigerator for a few hours before cutting. Once cool, remove from baking dish and cut into desired size. Store in airtight container or bags.

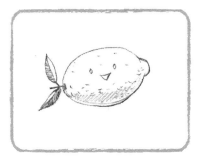

Sweet Tooth Upgrades

Sweet Mochi Rice is made by the pressing of sweet brown rice. If you love warm pastries, then don't miss out on this sweet treat! Look for MOCHI at your favorite health food store.

Vegan & Sugar Free Ice Cream

Make your own:

1. Get some fresh fruit
2. Blend
3. Freeze a little
4. Stir, and then blend again to make a nice consistency.

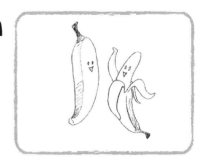

Banana "Ice Cream" (Yo'nana'gert)

* 2 medium/large bananas
* 3 Medjool dates OR 3-5 drops of vanilla stevia
* 1/4 - 1/2 cup almond milk
* 1/4 tsp cinnamon

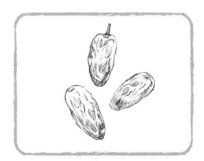

Directions:

1. Freeze bananas.
2. Place bananas, dates, cinnamon, and 1/4 cup of almond milk in a blender and blend until smooth.
3. SLOWLY add more almond Milk until desired consistency.

Chocolate Chia 'Pudding'

* 1 large avocado (ripe)
* 1/2 cup soaked raw organic cashews
* 1/2 cup nut milk
* 1/2 cup pitted dates (Medjool)
* 1/4 cup grade B maple syrup (or 1/8 tsp stevia)
* 1/3 cup raw cacao powder (no sugar, no artificial sweeteners)
* 1 tsp cinnamon
* 1 tsp ground chia seeds
* 1/2 - 1 tsp pure vanilla extract or powder
* 1/8 tsp Celtic Sea Salt

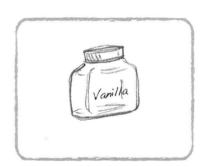

Directions:

1. Put all ingredients into a blender and blend.
2. Variation: add 3/4 cup of pure organic pumpkin, sweet potato, or your favorite squash.
3. For a 'tapioca' type texture: combine 2 TBSP chia seeds with purified water.
4. Mix vigorously for 1 minute.
5. Let sit and then mix again every 2 minutes for 10 minutes.
6. Hand mix into the 'pudding'.

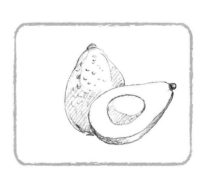

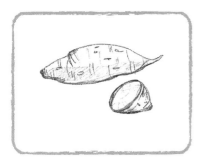

Sweet Potato Pie

Crust

* 1 cup gluten free organic oats
* ¼ buckwheat flour
* ½ cup walnuts / pecans
* ¼ mixture chia/water
* ¼ coconut oil
* 1 tsp Celtic sea salt (to taste)

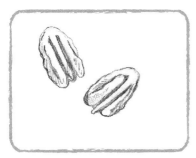

Directions:

1. Slightly roast oats, buckwheat flour, walnuts and pecans.
2. Lightly pulse in blender or food processor.
3. Add chia, coconut oil and salt.
4. Blend together and then push into a lightly oiled baking pan.
5. You can pre-bake the crust for 15 minutes before adding filling.

Filling

* 2 ¼ cups sweet potato
* ½ cup coconut sugar
* ¼ cup almond milk
* 1tsp coconut oil
* ¼ cup grade B maple syrup
* 3 tsp arrowroot
* 4 tsp chia gel (1/2 tsp chia, 4 tsp water)
* 2 tsp vanilla
* 2 tsp pumpkin spice
* ½ tsp Celtic sea salt (to taste)

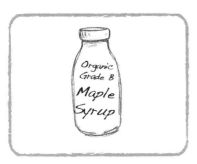

Directions:

1. Preheat Oven to 350 degrees.
2. Blend ingredients together in a food processor or by hand or hand-held blender.
3. Pour batter into crust.
4. Bake at 350 for 25 minutes or until desired taste.

Vegan Sweet Cream

* Avocado
* 1 cup soaked (1 hour) raw cashews
* 2-5 drops of favorite liquid stevia (such as vanilla)

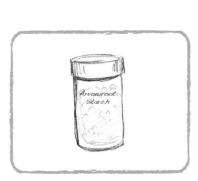

Directions:

1. Place all ingredients in blender.
2. Blend until smooth.

Sweet Potato Chips

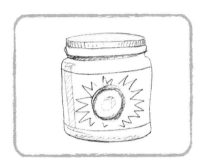

* 1 medium sweet potato
* 2 TBSP coconut oil
* Celtic Sea Salt and spices to taste

Directions:

1. Try different organic vegetables for the chips: carrots, turnips, zucchini, different squashes, etc. For a sweeter chip, try apples!

2. Preheat oven to 400 degrees. Wash sweet potato (peel sweet potato - optional).

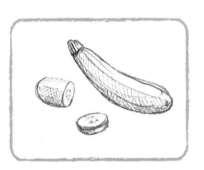

3. With a mandolin slicer OR with a sharp knife cut into very thin pieces (a mandolin will be much easier for this).

4. In a mixing bowl, combine melted coconut oil, sea salt and favorite spices (for hot, add a little cayenne pepper or try smoked paprika).

5. Add the thinly sliced sweet potatoes to the mixture. With your hands, begin to mix so that each 'chip' is coated with oil and spice.

6. Spread out on a cookie sheet or use parchment paper placed on top of a cookie sheet.

7. Bake for 5-8 minutes.

8. Flip the chips and bake for another 3-5 minutes.

9. Check every few minutes so they do not burn. The size of the 'chip' determines how quickly they will bake.

Baby Food Recipes

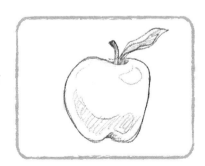

Look for the organic, nothing-added baby food. It's still heated and pasteurized, but it's hopefully pure without anything added. Remember to always read ingredients.

Examples of Organic Baby food found in jars:

Sweet Potatoes, Carrots, Bananas, Peas, Prunes, Apricots, etc. Mixtures of vegetables, fruits, and even grains and poultry

When in a pinch, get these simple items. This is a good starter for a sauce (such as sweet potatoes) if you don't want to bake and puree!!!! If you need pumpkin for a recipe, get organic pumpkin baby food in a glass jar (instead of canned pumpkin).

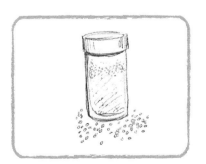

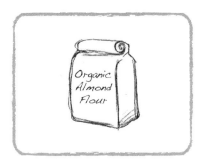

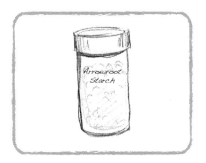

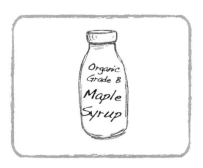

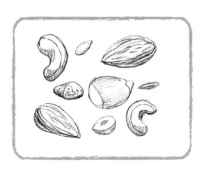

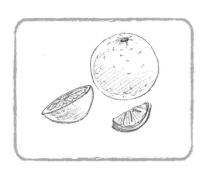

Almond Biscotti

* 1-½ cup organic almond flour (alternative: use finely ground organic almonds))

* 1 TBSP arrowroot powder

* ½ tsp aluminum-free baking soda

* ¼ tsp Celtic Sea Salt or Himalayan Salt

* ¼ cup organic maple syrup
  (or coconut sugar or coconut nectar)

* ¼ cup chopped organic almonds or other nuts/seeds

* 3 TBSP freshly squeezed, organic orange juice

* 2 TBSP organic orange zest

* ¼ cup cacao powder, cacao nibs OR unsweetened dark chocolate chips

Directions:

1. Preheat oven to 350F degrees.

2. Use a large glass baking dish or cookie sheet, and line with natural wax or parchment paper

3. First, wash the organic orange and with a fine grater, then grate the orange. Grate until you see the pith (white stuff) then turn over the orange to the other side and if needed, grate more. Use a hand held juicer, reamer, or blender to juice the rest of the orange.

4. Using a food processor, add almond flour, arrowroot powder, aluminum-free baking soda and Upgraded Salt.

5. Combine ingredients well in food processor or mix by hand.

6. Bring food processor to a very slow speed or if you don't have that option, use the pulse button and slowly add in maple syrup (or Upgraded sweetener of choice), orange zest, and orange juice. If you don't have a food processor, mix by hand.

7. Use the slow speed or pulse until a dough-like consistency forms.

8. Remove the dough from the food processor and hand mix in the chopped almonds/nuts/seeds and cacao powder, nibs, or dark chocolate.

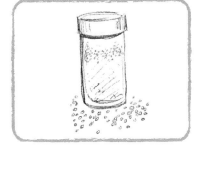

9. Dampen your hands and then on wax or parchment paper, create a log with the dough - approximately 2" inches high.

10. Bake at 350 degrees for 15-20 minutes or until firm to the touch or lightly brown.

11. Remove from the oven and cool for about1 hour. Remember to turn off oven! After cooled, cut into ½"- ¾" slices. Use a very sharp knife and cut on the diagonal.

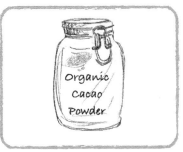

12. Preheat oven to 250F degrees. Spread out the slices on your dish or cookie sheet (with the CUT SIDE DOWN).

13. Bake at 250F for 10 minutes.

14. Turn over slices and bake for an additional 10 minutes.

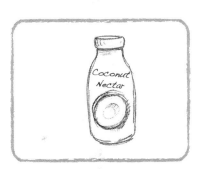

15. Then TURN OFF THE OVEN **but do not open it**!

16. Let slices sit in the oven for approximately two hours until cool and crunchy.

These biscotti are so delicious! Again, play with the ingredients.

Add ingredients you love and leave out the ones you don't like.

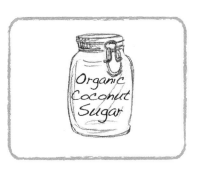

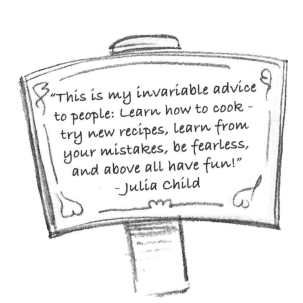

"This is my invariable advice to people: Learn how to cook - try new recipes, learn from your mistakes, be fearless, and above all have fun!"
— Julia Child

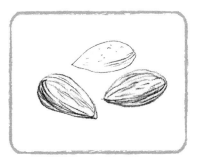

APPENDIX B - REFERENCES

Books & Journals
Cherniske, S. (1998) Caffeine Blues: Wake Up to the Hidden Dangers of America's #1 Drug. New York, NY: Warner Books/Hatchette Book Group.

Cousens, G. (2003) Rainbow Green Live Food Cuisine. Berkeley, CA: North Atlantic Books.

Fallon, S. & Enig M. (2003). Nourishing Traditions: The Cookbook that Challenges Politically Correct Nutrition and the Diet Dictocrats. Warsaw, IN: Newtrends Publishing, Inc.

Monte, W. C. (1984). Aspartame: Methanol and the Public Health. Journal of Applied Nutrition, 36(1), 42-54.

Pitchford, P. (2002). Healing With Whole Foods: Asian Traditions and Modern Nutrition (3rd Edition). Berkeley, CA: North Atlantic Books.

Rosenthal, J. (2008). Integrative Nutrition: Feed Your Hunger For Health and Happiness. New York, NY: Integrative Nutrition Publishing.

Stanchich, L. (1989). Power Eating Program: You Are How You Eat. Healthy Products, Inc.

Turner, K. (2002). The Self-Healing Cookbook: Whole Foods To Balance Body, Mind and Moods (9th Edition): Vashon, WA: Earthtones Press.

Yoshiko, F., Masanori, H., Okada, M., Hayashi, S., Nabeno, Y., Osawa, T., & Michitaka, N. (2008). Lemon Polyphenols Suppress Diet-induced Obesity by Up-Regulation of mRNA Levels of the Enzymes Involved in β-Oxidation in Mouse White Adipose Tissue. Journal of Clinical Biochemistry & Nutrition, 43(3), 201–209.

Websites
Addiction (July 8, 2014). Your Brain on Sugar. http://www.addictiontreatmentmagazine.com/addiction/food-addiction/brain-sugar/

Care2 (2015). 10 Benefits and Uses For Miso. http://www.care2.com/greenliving/10-benefits-and-uses-for-miso.html

Chris Kresser (2015). Harmful or Harmless: Guar Gum, Locust Bean Gum, and More. http://chriskresser.com/harmful-or-harmless-guar-gum-locust-bean-gum-and-more

Dr. Mark Hyman (January 8, 2015). 5 Reasons Most Diets Fail (and How to Succeed). http://drhyman.com/blog/2014/05/26/5-reasons-diets-fail-succeed/

Environmental Working Group (2015). Dirty Dozen and Clean Fifteen. http://www.ewg.org/foodnews/summary.php

Harvard Health Publications Blog (January 8, 2014). Mindfulness meditation may ease anxiety, mental stress. http://www.health.harvard.edu/blog/mindfulness-meditation-may-ease-anxiety-mental-stress-201401086967

Herb Wisdom (2014-2015). Lemons (Fruit). http://www.herbwisdom.com/herb-lemon.html

Kripalu (May 29, 2013). Daily Stress Relief: Shake It Off! http://kripalu.org/blog/thrive/2013/05/29/daily-stress-relief-shake-it-off/

Mercola (1997-2015). Bad to the Last Drop: Refiners Squeeze Dangerous Additives from Corn [Report]. http://www.mercola.com/Downloads/bonus/danger-of-corn-syrup/report.aspx

Mercola (1997- 2015). Probiotics for Your Gut Health. http://probiotics.mercola.com/probiotics.html

Mercola (June 28, 2005). The Surprising Toxic Effects of Vegetable Oils. http://articles.mercola.com/sites/articles/archive/2005/06/28/vegetable-oils.aspx

Mercola (October 13, 2009). Artificial Sweeteners – More Dangerous Than You Ever Imagined. http://articles.mercola.com/sites/articles/archive/2009/10/13/artificial-sweeteners-more-dangerous-than-you-ever-imagined.aspx

Mercola (August 10, 2010). The Cholesterol Myth That Is Harming Your Health. http://articles.mercola.com/sites/articles/archive/2010/08/10/making-sense-of-your-cholesterol-numbers.aspx?i_cid=cse-tbd-cholesterol-content

Mercola (September 9, 2012). The Amazing Similarities Between this Toxic Sugar and Alcohol. http://articles.mercola.com/sites/articles/archive/2012/09/09/ethanol-alcohol-and-fructose.aspx

Mercola (March 22, 2014). First Case Study to Show Direct Link Between Alzheimer's and Aluminum Toxicity. http://articles.mercola.com/sites/articles/archive/2014/03/22/aluminum-toxicity-alzheimers.aspx

Rodale News (2009-2013). 7 Hidden Dangers of Artificial Sweeteners. http://www.rodalenews.com/dangers-artificial-sweeteners

SF Gate (2015). Healthy Eating: Four Classes of Digestive Enzymes. http://healthyeating.sfgate.com/four-classes-digestive-enzymes-9941.html

Tasty Yummies (2010-2015). 10 Benefits to Drinking Warm Lemon Water Every Morning. http://tasty-yummies.com/2013/03/18/10-benefits-to-drinking-warm-lemon-water-every-morning/

Truth in Labeling (March 2014). Names of ingredients that contain processed free glutamic acid (MSG). http://www.truthinlabeling.org/hiddensources.html

University of Texas Health Science Center, San Antonio (June 27, 2011). Related studies point to the illusion of the artificial [Press release]. http://uthscsa.edu/hscnews/singleformat2.asp?newID=3861

Appendix / Index

A

Acai 161
Acidic stomach 71
acidity 68
ADD 68, 71
Addiction 226
Addictive 68, 95
Add-Ins/Upgrades 28
ADHD 68, 71
Advertising 69
Agave 77, 86
Alcoholism 68, 71
All calories are NOT the same 222
Allergies 71
Almond Biscotti 262
Almond Flour 161
Almond Milk 234
Almonds 161
Aloe Vera 161
Alzheimer's 68, 71
Amaranth 161
Amaranth Veggie Patties 241
Americano 30
Animal-Based Fats 59
Apple Butter 248
Apple Cider Vinegar 31, 162
Apple Cider Vinegar Tonic Drink 31
Apple Pie (Breakfast) 134
Apples 162
Applesauce 84
Appropriate Movement 229
Apricot puree 84
Are you dehydrated 36
Are you willing to Upgrade? 71
Arrowroot Starch 162
Artificial Flavorings 94
Artificial Sweeteners 73, 74, 75
Artificial sweeteners are TOXIC
    CHEMICALS 73
Artificial Sweeteners create WEIGHT
    Gain 74
Artificial sweeteners Desensitize taste
    buds 73
Artificial Sweeteners found in 73
Asparagus 162
Asparagus Soup 102
Aspartame 74
Aspartame, symptoms 74
Avocado & Kale Salad 255
Avocado Lemon Dill Dressing 253
Avocado Mushroom Sauce 252
Avocados 101, 162

B

Baby Food Recipes 261
Baby Formula 97
Baby-Stepology 8, 13
Baby Steps 17, 19, 22, 26, 33, 45, 51, 55,
    65, 72, 80, 87, 98, 103, 113, 119,
    122, 126, 148, 157, 159, 190, 193,
    206, 215, 225
Baked Amaranth Veggie Patties 241
Baking Powder 153
Banana "Ice Cream" 259
Bananas 84, 162
Barley Malt 86
Basic Vegetable Broth 240
Basil 162
Basmati Brown Rice 163
Beans/Legumes 62, 163, 244
Bean Spread 246
Beans Soaking Time: 244
Be gentle and kind with yourself! 82
Bell Peppers 163
Benefits of Movement 217
Benefits of Sauerkraut 125
Benefits of supplemental enzymes 121
Beverages 142
    How to Upgrade 146
Beverage UPGRADE Chart 143
Beverage Upgrades 148
Binders 156
    Thickeners 155
Biscotti 262
Black Strap Molasses 84
Bloated 120
Blood-Sugarology 9, 101
Blood Sugar Stability 39
Blood Sugar Stabilization 114, 222
Blueberries 163
Brain Fog 71
Brazil Nuts 163
Breakfast 78, 112
Breakfast Chia 29
Breakfast Foods , 133
Breakfast Options 158, 195
Broccoli 163
Brown Rice 163
Brown Sugar 86
Brussels Sprouts 164
Buckwheat Flour 164
Buckwheat Grouts 164
Budget 187
Burdock 164
Butter 59, 153
Butternut Squash Soup 238

C

Cacao Butter, Paste & Powder 164
Cacao Nibs 164
"Caesar" Salad 255
Caffeine Habit 145
Cancer 71, 192
Canola oil 92
Carbohydrates 156
    Fast Carbs / Slow Carbs & Fruit Carbs
    116
    Slow Carbs 117
Cardamom 165
Cardamom Almond Cookies 258
Carob Powder 165
Carrot Butter 248
Carrots 165
Cashew Cream Frosting - Vegan 258
Cashews 165
Cauliflower 165
Cayenne Pepper 165
Celeriac 165
Celery 166
Celery Root 165
Celtic Sea Salt 31, 166
Chamomile Tea 32
Cherries 166
Chia Seeds 29, 101, 166
Chickpeas 166
Childhood Memories 20
Chips - Sweet Potato 261
Chocolate Chia 'Pudding' 259
Chocolate Chip Cookies 151
Cholesterol and its bad rap 60
Chronic Fatigue 71
Cilantro 166
Cinnamon 28, 166
Coconut Crystals 167
Coconut Flakes 167
Coconut Flour 167
Coconut Milk 167
Coconut Nectar 77, 167
Coconut Oil 30, 167
Coconut Sugar 77, 83, 167
Coconut Sugar or Coconut Palm Sugar
    83
Coffee Drinks 30
Coffee - No-Withdrawal Example 145
Cold-Pressed 92
Comforting Foods 40
Commercials 69
Community 39
Community functions 69
Condiments 138
Condiments to Upgrade 105

Cookies 151, 258, 262
Cooking Hints 185
Cookware 192
Corn 90
Corn Oil 92
Cranberries 84
Craveology 8, 35
Craving Fast Carbs 44
Craving Fried/Oily Foods 44
Craving Q's 43
Cravings 36, 40, 44, 131
Cravings, common causes of 38
Cravings, feelings 42
Cravings, Messages 35
Cravings, Patterns 37
Cravings, reasons 37
Cravings, Salt 44
Craving Sugar 44
Cream - Vegan 260
Creamy 109
Creamy Asparagus Soup 102
Create Your Own Sauces and Spreads 108
Crock-Pot/Slow Cooker 237
Cucumbers 167
Cumin Avocado Dressing 196, 254
Current events 39

D

Daikon Radish 168
Dairy 88, 155
Dairy Upgrades 135
Dandelion Greens 168
Dates 83, 171
Date Sugar 84
Date Syrup 77
Dehydrating 48
Dehydration 38, 47, 205
Dehydration, signs 47
Delegate Your Issues 214
Dementia 68
Depression 68, 71
Desert island 75
Detox 76
Detox from Sugar Without Biting Off Someone's Head 76
Dextrose 94
Diabetes 68, 71, 74
Diet 5
Diets 13
Diet soda INCREASES your risk of diabetes 74
Digestion 121

Digestive issues 95
Dijon Mustard 250
Dill 168
Don't Judge a Product by its Nutritional Facts 54
Dressing 140
Dried Fruits 77
Drink Purified Water 48, 228
Dulse Flakes 168

E

Easy Upgrades to get you started 131
Eggs 155
Endless Curiosity 15
Energizing Drink 179
Energizing Snacks 115
Energy 178
Enzymes 120, 121
Enzymes that help digest your food 120
Essential Omega-3 Fatty Acids 63
Excellent enzymatic foods to try 121
Excess Weight 71
Expeller-pressed 92

F

Famous Failures 35
FAST Carb Conversions 156
Fast Carbs 116
Fast Carbs / Slow Carbs / Fruit Carbs 116, 156
Fast Carbs to Upgrade 116
Fast Carbs vs Slow Carbs 44
Fat-Free or Low-Fat Foods 78
Fatigue 68, 71
Fats 93, 102, 111
Fermented 89
Fermented Vegetables 123
Fiber 102
Fiber, Protein & Fat 104
Fibromyalgia 68, 71
Fill Up Faster and Stay Satisfied 64
Finance$ 214
Flavor 64
Flax Seeds 101, 168
Florida Cane Crystals 86
Flour 152
Flu 68
Food Addiction 226
Food Coloring 94
Food Combinations to Help Harmonize Mood & Stabilize Blood Sugar 101

Food education 69
Food Item / Side Effects 186
Food Marketing 69
Food/Mood Journal 126
Food Plan 194
Food Prep Guide 191
Frankenfoods 70, 73, 82, 88
Freshly squeezed juices 85
Frozen 57
Frozen Meals 184
Fruit 77, 78
Fruit Carbs 116
Fruit Juices & Smoothies 178

G

Garam Masala 168
Garbanzo Bean Flour 168
Garlic 169
Gentle Yoga 209
Ghee 169
Ginger 169
Gingered Black Beans 245
Ginger-Garlic Sauce 252
Give yourself an Alternative 82
Gluten-Free 91
Gluten-Free Grains 62, 91
Glutenous Whole Grains 62
Gluten sensitivity 91
GMO 58
Going Out - Your Third Place 187
Goji Berries 169
Golden Milk Recipe 236
Gotta Go Bag 118
Grade B Maple Syrup 77, 83
Granola Bars I 256
Granola Bars II 257
Grapefruit 61, 77, 169
Gratitude 18, 216
Green Stevia Powder 77, 83
Green Tea 32, 171
Grocery store 55
Guacamole 249
Gums 156
    Thickeners 155

H

Hazelnuts 169
Headache 24
Headaches 95, 205
Healing Foods 161
Healingology 10, 161
Hemp Seeds 169

Appendix / Index

Herbicides 58
Hidden Sugar 70
High fructose corn syrup (HFCS) 77
Himalayan Salt 31, 173
Holidays 38, 69
Hollandaise Sauce 107
Honey, Raw & Unprocessed 170
Hormone Issues 71
Hormones 38
Horseradish Root 170
Hospitals 69
Hot Chocolate 30
How To Set Goals 20
Hummus 245
Hunger, Mouth vs Belly 228
Hydrating 48
Hydrogenated 92
Hypoglycemic 68, 71

I

I CAN List 181, 182, 183
Ice Cream 135, 259
Ingredient Conversions 152
    Baking Powder 153
    Butter 153
    Dairy 155
    Eggs 155
    FAST Carb Conversions 156
    Flour 152
    Hydrogenated Oils 154
    Margarine 154
    Refined Sugar Upgrades 154
    Thickeners 155
Ingredientologist 67
Ingredientology 8, 53
Ingredientology is simple 53
Ingredients 41, 53, 54, 70, 76, 97, 228
Instead of Cereal 158
Introduction 4
It's all about the ... 213
It's all about the SAUCE! 106

J

Job/Career/Work 38
Juices 85
Junk Food, Office 27

K

Kale 170
Kefir 123

Kelp 170
Ketchup 250
Kid's cereal 97
Kimchi 123
Kitchen Sanctuary 189
Kiwi 170
Kombucha 123

L

Lack of Movement 39
Lacuma 84
Latte 30
Laugh 213
Leafy Greens 61
Learn How to Increase Energy With
    Nourishing Foods 161
Lemon 77
Lemon Benefits 49
Lemons 170
Limes 170
Liquid Stevia 85
Liver 77
Low glycemic 77
Lucuma 171
Lunch & Dinner Options 196

M

Maca 171, 236
Macadamia Nuts 171
Magic Trio Combination 101, 104
Make Your Own Dressing 140
Malls 69
Maple Syrup 83, 171
Margarine 60, 154
Margarine WARNING 60
Matcha Green Tea Powder 171
'Mayo' Dressing 251
Meals 136
Meal Upgrades 136
Medical Issues 57
Meditation 208
Medjool Dates 171
Mesquite Powder 171
Millet "Mashed Potatoes" 242
Mineral Rich Salts 60
Minimally processed 92
Miso Paste 123, 172
Miso - Sesame Butter Dip 254
Mocha 30
Modified 92
Money-Saving Tips 57

"Morning Apple Pie" 134
Morning Rice 232
Morning Smoothie Options 158
Most important meal of the day 112
Movement & Exercise 216
Movement Options 217
Movement Worries 218
Moving Meditation 208
MSG 95
MSG, Some of the names of MSG 95
Mushrooms 172
Mustard 250
My Upgrade List 150

N

Names for soy 89
Natural Flavorings 94
Naturally Sweet and Nurturing Foods
    228
NON-GMO 58, 89
Not-So-Sweet Effects of Artificial
    Sweeteners 74
Nourishing Animal FATS 111
Nourishing Fats and Oils 59
Nourishing Foods 59
    Index of Healing Foods 161
Nourishing Plant Based Fats 102, 111
Nourishing Protein 63
Nut Milk 234
Nut Milk Variations 235
Nutrient Deficient Foods 38
Nutrient Fiber 102
Nutritional Facts 53, 54, 97
Nutritional Yeast 172
Nuts and Seeds 62, 96, 121
Nutty 109

O

Oats 172
Obesity 68, 71
Office Junk Food 27
Offices 69
Oil 92
Olive Oil 59, 172
Omega-3s 63
Onion Family 61
Onions 61, 172
Orange Zest 85
Organic Extra Virgin Olive Oil 172
Organics 56
Organics & Future Generations 56

Organic Shopping Tips 187
Organics Shopping Tips 57
Organization 188
Othman, Ayu 273
Overnight Oats 232

P

Palm Sugar 77
Pancakes - Grain Free 231
Papayas 121
Paprika 172
Parasites 192
Passion 211
PASSION - Engage in something you
  love! 229
Peaches 173
Peanut Caution 63
Peas 173
Pecans 173
Peppermint Tea 32
Periodontal disease 68, 71
Pesticides 56, 58
Pie - Sweet Potato 260
Pineapples 121, 173
Ping-Pong 4
Pistachios 173
Plant-Based 59
Plant-Based Nourishing FATS 111
PLU 58
Pomegranate 173
Popcorn 90
Portion Control? 157
Pre-diabetes 68
Prepare for Eating 224
Prepare for Sleep 202
Price, Dr. Weston A. 71
Probiotic Foods 64, 122
Processed & Packaged Foods - a.k.a.
  Frankenfoods 70
Produce Labels & Stickers 58
Produce Prep Tips 191
Protein 102
Protein Powder 134
Protein Shakes 97, 134
'Pudding' - Chocolate Chia 259
Pumpkin 174
Pumpkin Seeds 174

Q

Quality Protein 102
Questionable Sweeteners 86

Quinoa 174
Quinoa Bean Burgers 241
Quinoa Tabouli 243
Quirky or Perky ? 144
Quote
  Hippocrates 161

R

Raspberries 174
Raw 121
Raw and SPROUTED Nuts and Seeds
  121
Raw Fruits 121
Raw Fruits and Vegetables 121
Raw Honey 77, 83
READ Ingredients 41
Rebellion 20
Rebellious 20
Recipe Alterations 150
Recipes
  Almond Biscotti 262
  Almond Milk 234
  Amaranth Veggie Patties 241
  Apple Butter 248
  Apple Cider Vinegar Tonic Drink 31
  Avocado & Kale Salad 255
  Avocado Lemon Dill Dressing 253
  Avocado Mushroom Sauce 252
  Baby Food 261
  Banana "Ice Cream" 259
  Basic Vegetable Broth 240
  Beans 244
  Bean Spread 246
  Beans Soaking Time 244
  Beverages 142
  Breakfast Chia 29
  Breakfast Options 158
  Butternut Squash Soup 238
  Cardamom Almond Cookies 258
  "Ceasar" Salad 255
  Chocolate Chia 'Pudding' 259
  Chocolate Chip Cookies 151
  Condiments 138
  Creamy Asparagus Soup 102
  Crock-Pot/Slow Cooker 237
  Cumin Avocado Dressing 254
  Dijon Mustard 250
  Dressing 140
  Gingered Black Beans 245
  Ginger-Garlic Sauce 252
  Golden Milk Recipe 236
  Granola Bars 256

Hollandaise Sauce 107
Hot Chocolate 30
Hummus 245
Ice Cream 259
Ingredient Conversions 152
Ketchup 250
'Mayo' Dressing 251
Meal Upgrades 136
Millet "Mashed Potatoes" 242
Miso - Sesame Butter Dip 254
"Morning Apple Pie" 134
Morning Rice 232
Mustard 250
My Upgrade List 150
Nut Milk 234
Nut Milk Variations 235
Overnight Oats 232
Popcorn 90
Protein Shakes 134
Quinoa Bean Burgers 241
Quinoa Tabouli 243
Recipe Alterations 150
Refined Sugar Upgrades 154
Rice Drink 'Horchata' 235
Root Soup 239
Sauerkraut 124
Seed Cheeze 247
Simple Grain Free Pancakes 231
Simple Guacamole 249
Slow Cooked Grains 237
S'mores 83
Snacks 115, 137
Steel Cut Oatmeal 233
Stevia 85
Sweet Carrot Butter 248
Sweet Potato Chips 261
Sweet Potato Pie 260
Tahini Dressing 196
Tangy Rice Pilaf 240
The Crock Pot Has Gone Nuts! 237
Trail Mix 257
Vegan Cashew Cream Frosting 258
Vegan Cashew Ranch Dressing 253
Vegan Cheeze 246
Vegan Egg Substitute 231
Vegan 'Hollandaise' Sauce 249
Vegan 'Mayo' 251
Vegan Sour Cream 248
Vegan Sweet Cream 260
Veggie Pizza 243
Worcestershire-ish Sauce 107
Zucchini Pasta 242
Red Lentils 174
Reduce Inflammation 121

Appendix / Index

Reduce Stress 229
Refreshing 109
Relationships 39
Release the Diet Mentality 110
Restful Sleep Rituals 201
Rice Drink 'Horchata' 235
Root Soup 239
Rose Hips 174
Rosemary 174

S

Sale/Coupons 187
Salt 94
Salty 108
Satisfaction Chart 21
Sauce 107
Sauerkraut 123, 124
Schools 69
Scream and Shout About It! 212
Seasons 38
Seed Cheeze 247
Self-Acceptance 221
Self-Kindness 221
Self-Talk or Self-Sabotage? 221
Sesame Seeds (Tahini) 175
Shake Shake Shake 212
Shallots 175
Shopping & Cooking Strategies for
    Successful Upgrading 181
Side Effects of Refined Sugar 68
Simple Food/Mood Journal 127
Simple, no-equipment exercises for
    your home and office 218
Sing your favorite song 213
Sitting Forward Fold 209
Sitting Lateral Stretch 210
Sitting Twist 209
Skin irritations 95
Skin issues 71
Sleep 229
Slippery Elm 175
Slow Carbs 117
Slow Cooked Grains 237
Slow Cooker 192
Smoothie/ Protein Powder 158
Snack Bar 97
Snack OPTIONS 198
Snacks 79, 103, 114, 115, 137
Snacks & Blood Sugar Stabilization 114
Snack Upgrades
    Snacks 137
Soda 68, 74

Sour Cream - Vegan 248
Sour or Zesty 108
Soy 89
Soy Alternative Upgrades 89
Soybean Oil 92
Spaghetti Squash 175
Spices 64, 85
Spinach 175
Spirulina 175
Sprouts 121, 175
Sprouts, grow your own 184
Stabilize blood sugar 101
STABLE blood sugar graph 114
Steel Cut Oatmeal 233
Stevia 85
Stevia, Green Leaf or Powder 83, 176
Story
    A depressed man 35
    Purple unicorn 36
Strawberries 176
Stress 39, 79
Stress Relief 207
Stretch Breaks 208
Sucanat 86
Successology 10, 181
Sucralose 86
Sugar 67, 70, 76, 79
Sugar, Addiction 76
Sugar and Food Addiction 226
Sugar Kiss 66
Sugar Questions 79
Sugar, Refined and Artificial 78
Sugar Symptoms 71
Sugar & The Dangers of Food Market-
    ing 69
Sugar, Upgraded 83
Sugar, Upgrades 154
Summary of Baby Steps 228
Sunflower Seeds 176
Support and Help! 229
Sweet Carrot Butter 248
Sweetened Fruit Juice 86
Sweetened Iced Tea Options 142
Sweeteners, Upgraded 83
Sweet, make your own sauce 108
Sweetology & Frankenology 9, 67
Sweet Potato Chips 261
Sweet Potatoes 176
Sweet Potato Pie 260
Sweet vegetables 78
Symptoms 24, 71, 74
    Detox signs 76
Symptoms Chart 25

T

Tahini 175, 176
Tahini Dressing 196, 254
Take a deep breath 207
Talk to someone positive 213
Tangy Rice Pilaf 240
Taste/Leftovers 38
Tea 32
Teflon 192
Testimonials 7, 272
    Susan, New Mexico 24
    Tina 207
The Baby Step Approach 13
The Banana Versus the Pancake 81
The Crock Pot Has Gone Nuts! 237
The Importance of Reading Ingredients
    53
The root of her headaches? 205
The Scary on Artificial Sweeteners -
    a.k.a. Frankenfoods 73
The Sticky on Gums a.k.a. - Binders
    156
The Void 38
The Why Upgrade List... 186
Thickeners 155
Tips For Whole Body Wellness 201
Tomatoes 176
Tonic Drink - Apple Cider Vinegar 31
Tooth decay 71
Toxic and Fake Food-Like-Stuff 88
TOXIC CHEMICALS 73
Toxic Fats 93
Toxic Ingredients 94
Toxic Oils to be Avoided 92
Trail Mix 257
Truth In Labeling 95
Turmeric 28, 176

U

Umami 95
Understanding What's In YOUR Food
    67
Understand Your Food Cravings &
    Their Hidden Messages 35
Understand Your Food, Understand
    Your Mood 9, 126
Unicorn 36
Unplug and get connected with nature
    and real people 214
Unrefined 92
Unsatisfied 34
UNSTABLE blood sugar graph 114

Upgrade 5, 40, 76, 229
Upgraded Beverages 142
UPGRADED Fats 93
Upgraded Oils 92
Upgraded Recipe Example: 151
Upgraded Sweeteners 83
Upgrade from Toxic & Artificial Foods 97
Upgradeology 6, 10, 131
Upgrades 131
Upgrades for Refined Sugar & Artificial Sweeteners 77
Upgrades from FrAnkEnfoods 88
Upgrades Options 132
Upgrade Your Cravings 44
Upgrade Your Family & Get Them on Board 157
Upgrade Your Favorite Drink 143

V

Vanilla Bean Powder 177
Vegan Cashew Cream Frosting 258
Vegan Cashew Ranch Dressing 253
Vegan Cheeze 246
Vegan Egg Substitute 231
Vegan 'Hollandaise' Sauce 249
Vegan 'Mayo' 251
Vegan Sour Cream 248
Vegan Sweet Cream 260
Vegetable Oil is EXTREMELY mis-leading! 92
Vegetables 60
Veggie Pizza 243
Vision problems 71
Visual Triggers 39

W

Walnuts 177
Water 46
Watermelon 177
Water Questions 50
Water Tips 49
Weight Gain 74
Weight Release 220
Wellnessology 11, 201
Wheat 91
Wheat Alternatives 91
Wheatgrass Juice 177
White, Nicole 273
Whole Grains 62
Why Buy Organic? 57

Why The Upgrade Process Works 16
Why Upgrade 186
Willpower 35
Worcestershire-ish Sauce 107
Worry 42
Write it Down to Figure it Out 204

X

Xylitol 86

Y

Yacon Syrup 84, 177
Yoga 209
Yogurt 123
You ARE That Magic Pill! 201
Your furry friends 213
Your Nose 39

Z

Zucchini 177
Zucchini Pasta 242

Testimonials

"I have paid attention to my diet and exercise for many years. In January of 2014 I was told I was mildly pre diabetic. I began doing some research on line and at the library. I felt like I needed someone to talk to and learn from. The class I completed with Nicole White was very beneficial. I learned about substitutions for oils and sweeteners and the cook book Nicole provides has many delicious recipes. Nicole has helped me to refine my diet and empowered me to eat in an even more healthy way. It would have taken me months, if not years (if not never) to find all of the information Nicole provides through her talks and recipes. I am so thankful for having taken her class and would recommend her class to anyone who wants to understand about the foods we eat and how they affect every aspect of our life. Thank you again Nicole."
- Susan Skinner, NM

"Nicole - Your program has changed my life. You have enlightened me to examine all medications carefully, directed me in upgrading my foods, provided me with tasty alternatives, and helped me examine the stressors in my life that cause my blood sugars to rise. Thank you for all your help!!!"
- Jeanne M, UNM

"The vast amount of information provided within the workbook and during the sessions was phenomenal. There was so much valuable information and guidance provided throughout the classes. In my experience, Nicole is very dedicated to her students, ensuring that they get exactly what they need to ensure their success in making healthy changes. I've experienced more energy, better focus and healthier snack options since the program began. Some of the most beneficial parts of the program for me were the information provided, the food/mood journal, the cookbook and snack lists and Nicole's support. For me, the recorded sessions were extremely helpful and appreciated as I was quite busy and not able to attend the live sessions. I was able to go back at my leisure and review the sessions and continue at my own pace. I highly recommend this program. I believe this course is a life saver and provides all the tools you need to incorporate a healthier lifestyle. Thank You Nicole for putting together an amazing course!"
- Michelle Hale, UNM

"Participating in Nicole's Healing Diabetes Naturally class was a life-changing experience for me. It provided an opportunity to honestly examine how I was sabotaging my health and then provided numerous ideas, tools, and strategies to turn things around. And the class was just a beginning…revisiting the materials and resources provided, will help me to incorporate healthy new actions into my life in the future. Thank you, Nicole, for your nurturing guidance and for sharing your unending and practical knowledge about this subject".
- Terry N, Chico, CA

I began working with Nicole White in order to rid my body of toxic stress hormones. I learned natural ways to aid my system in recovering from a period in my life in which I experienced bad stress-related symptoms. Nicole really awakened my awareness as to what food I am putting in my body and its ultimate effects on my mood and energy. Since working with Nicole, I have switched to strictly organic food sources as my main nutrition. My body and mind are back to a better place! Nicole has great suggestions for any questions you may have regarding nutrition. I will carry this knowledge with me so that I can continue making the best choices for myself and my family nutrition-wise."
- Carolyn P, Albuquerque, NM

For more testimonials and information about the various programs that Nicole teaches, please visit: www.Upgradeology.com or www.NicoleWhiteWellness.com

About Nicole White

When I was eight, my mother put me on my first diet. At sixteen, I was a compulsive overeater and bulimic. While in college, I began to have severe wrist pains. Doctors called it carpal tunnel and they wanted me to have surgery. As I investigated more, I found that people who went through the surgery didn't necessarily get relief from this pain. An art teacher led me to an acupuncturist who gave me a list of foods to avoid. I took his suggestions, and got rid of the toxic foods and drinks. To my delight and surprise, the pain and inflammation disappeared! This began my journey into learning that food is medicine and artificial food contributes to inflammation and disease.

Even with that knowledge, I still put myself through extreme diets, which contributed to various eating disorders and that roller coaster of weight gain/weight loss/weight gain. I grew up with the message that thin was beautiful and successful and that overweight was ugly and lazy. Through my journey, I have worked to release those old beliefs and found that true well-being and self-acceptance are the ultimate success and beauty!

My journey has included becoming a Gentle Yoga and Meditation Instructor, Energy Healer, Certified Holistic Health Coach and Artist. It's my goal to share true wellness with my clients. I am a robust woman and embrace all that I am and release that which I am not. I no longer diet because I live the very concept of Upgradeology that I love to share and teach.

For additional information, about Group Classes, Private Coaching, and Upgradeology, please visit: www.Upgradeology.com or www.NicoleWhiteWellness.com.

About Ayu Othman

Ayu loves drawing, doodling and making eye candy for a living. She balances out her enjoyment of food and video games with her love for surfing waves, paddle sports, and other nature-y pursuits. You can check out more of Ayu's work at **www.ayuart.com**.

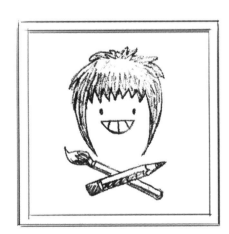

Made in the USA
San Bernardino, CA
28 June 2015